WITHDRAWN

Painbuster

Painbuster

- **A Breakthrough**

- **4-Step Program**

- **for Ending Pain**

JOHN M. STAMATOS, M.D.

with JANE O'BOYLE

HENRY HOLT AND COMPANY | NEW YORK

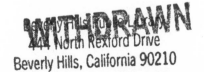

Henry Holt and Company, LLC
Publishers since 1866
115 West 18th Street
New York, New York 10011

Illustrations in chapter 5 are from *The American Physical Therapy Association Book of Body Maintenance and Repair* by Marilyn Moffat, PT, PhD, FAPTA, and Steve Vickery, illustrations by Terry Boles, © 1999 by Round Stone Press, Inc., and the American Physical Therapy Association. Reprinted by permission of Henry Holt and Company, LLC.

Illustrations on pages 29 and 63 are by Alesha Jutkofsky.

Library of Congress Cataloging-in-Publication Data

Stamatos, John M.
    Painbuster: a breakthrough 4-step program for ending pain / John M. Stamatos, with Jane O'Boyle.—1st ed.
        p.   cm.
    Includes index.
    ISBN 0-8050-6346-3 (hb)
    1. Chronic pain—Popular works.   2. Pain—Popular works.   3. Analgesia—Popular works.   I. O'Boyle, Jane.   II. Title.

RB127 .S7273 2001   00-049900
616'.0472—dc21

Henry Holt books are available for special promotions and premiums. For details contact: Director, Special Markets.

First Edition 2001

Printed in the United States of America

1   3   5   7   9   10   8   6   4   2

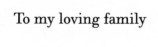
To my loving family

A Note to Readers

I have helped cure many pain patients, but this book is not a prescription for your specific pain syndrome. It is a model for you to follow with your physician. Please consult your own medical doctor, or one listed in the resources chapter, before embarking on any of these therapies.

Contents

Introduction

At any given moment, thirty-four million Americans suffer from chronic pain. Many have lower back pain or endure the pain of arthritis. Millions more suffer muscle and tissue injury, or painful debilitating illnesses like diabetes, fibromyalgia, or cancer. You or someone you know might easily be one of those pain sufferers. The policeman on medical leave for postsurgical pain from a repaired ruptured disc; the advertising executive with a nagging sports injury to her elbow; the bone cancer patient who repeatedly hears doctors tell him "there's nothing more we can do for your pain" and realizes he'll have to suffer for the rest of his life; the grandmother with arthritis who has been told "you simply must learn to live with the pain." Most chronic pain sufferers have spent years searching for relief without success. And as baby boomers enter middle age, while also caring for aging parents, there are more pain sufferers than ever before.

Pain can ruin your life. It can stop you from going to the movies because you can't sit still for two hours at a time. It can keep you from going to a museum because you can't stand, or walk, for very long either. Pain can distract you from your work, from taking proper care of your children, from concentrating on something as simple as reading or watching television. Chronic pain can depress you, frighten you, and make you irritable. Ultimately, pain can overwhelm you, and not only interfere with your normal life, but destroy it.

By the time a patient arrives in my office, he or she has usually spent weeks, months, or even years searching for relief. Most of my patients have been to several doctors and health-care providers who were not able, or willing, to help at all. Time and time again, they heard doctors tell them "you'll just have to learn to live with it." Many times, in a matter of days—sometimes even in just hours—my treatment methods can turn their lives around. I remember a patient, Brian D., a fifty-five-year-old lawyer who had suffered pain from a herniated disc for nearly four years. As he began his first day in years without pain, Brian telephoned to ask me an urgent question: "Why has it taken so long to find relief? How come no one told me about these cures sooner?"

There are several answers to these questions. One is that pain cannot be seen by a doctor, or in a test. Pain has never been given a satisfactory definition, even among medical professionals. Pain is a personal thing, different for every patient. As a totally subjective symptom, therefore, pain is often misdiagnosed and treated incorrectly. Some even believe that chronic pain is all in a patient's head, perhaps because so many people with pain are miserable. Many doctors don't want to deal with a patient's pain, because it is often a challenge to treat it successfully. Other doctors don't see pain management as a vital element to health care—it's not an emergency or a life-threatening illness. Managed-care organizations frequently delay or deny coverage outright for pain treatment. I once had a patient with a serious disorder known as reflex sympathetic dystrophy who said to me, with only a little sarcasm, that he wished he had cancer, so that his HMO would approve payment for the treatment. With so little respect even from the medical industry, it's little wonder pain patients feel guilty, as if they are responsible in some way for their condition.

Another reason people don't know enough about pain management is because, for many years, there were no effective treatments routinely available for pain. This is no longer true. Pain cures exist now, just as there are modern remedies for high blood pressure and heart disease. Many of these treatments are very new, so new that some doctors are not even aware of them. Even if the exact cause of your pain cannot be found, there are safe medications that work, and a program for you to follow that will heal you. I have refined these techniques in what I call the Painbuster program. Can you remember what it was like to be pain-free? This book will lead you back to a lifestyle you may have thought was gone forever.

The startling reality is that treating pain separately— as a disease to be cured in and of itself, and not merely as a symptom of some other illness—is a new idea in the medical community. Only in the last few years has pain management become a certification of the American Board of Medical Specialties. Even now, there are not many pain specialists in the United States, or anywhere, for that matter. But the medical treatment of pain is growing rapidly, in pain centers like the one where I work, and in the offices of internists and general practitioners across the country. People want an end to pain and, finally, so do their doctors.

I have been researching and treating pain my entire medical career. I have seen astounding medical advances in this specialty, especially in the last five years. About a year ago, I began to realize that my success with patients in New York could help people everywhere, if they were able to learn the Painbuster four-step program in a book like this. After all, not everyone can receive a doctor's referral to a pain center, much as I might wish they could. But everyone can ask his own doctor about these breakthroughs, some of which are beginning to become standard practice by general practitioners and internists in the treatment of pain. With this book, I hope to disseminate the latest and most current information, and to offer readers everywhere the tools to cure their chronic pain, once and for all.

The more options and tools you have, the better and faster you will be cured. I call the variety of treatment modalities an "armamentarium" against pain. That's an old military term from my days at Walter Reed Army Medical Center. But it's what I can offer readers and pain sufferers—an arsenal of specific, innovative treatment options. Let me help you dismantle the frustrating maze of dated information regarding pain treatment. No matter what your disease or condition, you can be pain-free for the rest of your life.

Painbuster

CHAPTER 1

A New Philosophy of Pain Management

There is a biological purpose to pain. It warns the body that something has gone wrong, such as a broken leg that needs attention or a sprained elbow that should be rested. It is a well-meaning diversion from a harmful lifestyle, forcing you to regroup and alter your habits. In fact, people who are born with congenital analgesia—the rare condition where one is unable to sense pain—live fairly short lives, because they repeatedly damage their bodies without knowing it. Even though pain may serve as the voice of nature, there is no purpose to long-lasting pain that enslaves you. The real challenge in today's medical world is to change the attitude of both doctors and patients toward pain management. Looking at the ways that pain was treated in the past helps us put our present attitude in perspective.

Throughout medical history, the relief of pain rarely entered the picture. A disease's *cure* was administered at any cost. On the contrary, pain was often regarded as a necessary element of healing. This theory was all a person had to cling to, throughout the centuries when there was no alternative. Without remedies, one had no choice but to endure it. On top of that, pain was also frequently misidentified as an emotion, as opposed to a sensation. Pain was the same as suffering, the emotion at the far end of the spectrum from pleasure. For hundreds of years, pain was omitted from the field of physiology, assigned instead to the realms of psychology or philosophy. In the mid-1600s, French philosopher René Descartes proposed that pain was a purely physical phenomenon, and not an emotion at all. Pain sensations, he said, were transmitted by nerves to the brain, like pulling a rope to ring a bell.

In 1965, psychologist Ronald Melzack and physiologist Patrick Wall proposed the gate-control theory—that pain impulses can be controlled in the spinal cord "gateway" before they get to the brain. Melzack and Wall scientifically proved that a person's emotions and thoughts greatly affected sensory nerve responses, that pain was more than just a physical stimulus response. In the late 1980s, Ronald Melzack found that pain is sometimes generated by the brain alone, even in the absence of stimulus on a sensory nerve. Melzack's studies showed that the brain operates a "neuromodule" to produce a pain experience, using input not only from sensory nerves, but from memory and mood. Stubbing your toe, for example, sends a pain signal up through the spinal cord gateway, and when it enters the brain, the signal joins up with a bunch of other signals— anticipation, memory, distractions, and mood. Together, this little group forms a toe-pain "neuromodule." For most people, the little grouping causes a small symphony of pain. For some, this group works together to extinguish pain instead: stubbing the toe might not even hurt such people. For others, according to Melzack, the toe-pain neuromodule can be triggered *even when the toe has not been stubbed.* A frightening chronic pain can be set off by a simple touch, memory, momentary fear, or growing frustration. A good example of this kind of pain is frostbite— someone who loses a finger to frostbite might find cold water painful, even many years later.

As a young doctor, I spent several years in the army, treating patients injured in Kuwait and Somalia. I didn't encounter the brutal battlefield conditions that war surgeons of previous generations did, but I saw plenty of pain. While I was still a resident at Walter Reed Army Medical Center in Washington, D.C., I came upon *The Management of Pain* by Dr. John J. Bonica at the hospital library. Weighing the impact of this on my medical career, I guess you could say his book changed my life. Bonica conceived and founded the first "pain center" back in the 1940s in Tacoma, Washington, and another one in Seattle a few years later. He was the first to treat pain as a disease all its own, using the multiple disciplines of neurology, orthopedics, psychology, and physical therapy, along with alternative therapies such as acupuncture. I was captivated by Bonica's ability to successfully treat a multitude of patients whose pain had previously confounded doctors for years. His book revealed how, with dedication and the proper tools, pain could be eliminated, even if the primary illness remained. This was revolutionary in the 1940s, and it was still considered revolutionary, fifty years later. Bonica, who died in 1993, inspired me to begin to meet the challenge of solving the most difficult cases, the worst, most chronic pains, including those where the cause of pain was never found.

I was one of the first residents at Walter Reed who decided to make pain management his specialty. As it happened, an army hospital was the perfect training facility for a young doctor in this new field. In addition to the routine cases such as obstetric pain and postsurgical pain, I confronted hundreds of cases of traumatic injury pain, nerve ailments, psychological disorders, phantom limb pain, post-traumatic stress disorder, and terminal illness.

Encouraged by the anesthesiology staff at Walter Reed, I began to use some of Bonica's pain-management techniques on hospital patients. I also started to implement newer technologies and medications, along with ancient and traditional pain-relieving methods such as acupuncture and exercise. I began to realize that combining treatments in distinct ways resolved many different kinds of pain. I also found that each pain case responded to its very own special combination of treatments. Sometimes I used a wide variety of methods simultaneously, and at other times the patient responded better if we used one at a time, rotating to a new method over the course of time. As Bonica had done, I enlisted help from the specialists in neurology, orthopedics, psychology, nutrition, and physical therapy to work together in each case. When one method of treatment failed to help a patient, we agreed together to move on to a new tactic. Eventually, we would forge a customized pain-relief program that worked for every patient. Working together, my colleagues and I devised the first pain-management program ever used for the United States Army. We never encountered a pain case we couldn't vastly improve or completely solve. We worked together like a team of detectives solving a case.

I like the image of a pain-management specialist as a sort of detective, using trial and error to root out clues and resolve a puzzling mystery. Medical detective skills are honed well if you are trained in anesthesiology, as I was. Anesthesiologists like to call themselves the second-best physicians in every specialty. Because of the variety of patients we treat, we have to know a lot about every aspect of medicine. Anesthesiologists are the second most knowledgeable cardiologists at the hospital. The second best oncologists, orthopedists, neurosurgeons, obstetricians, you name it. Whatever kind of pain exists, an anesthesiologist has to know how to treat it. We also have to know the properties of all medications people take, and how they interact with one another. Anesthesiologists have to know how to perform injections correctly, into every part of the human body, exactly where they need to be. Yes, we are the people who put patients to "sleep" during surgery but, more than that, we are the pain managers. We are the doctors who keep that patient *safe* during surgery, which can damage the body as much as being hit by a bus. We are the doctors who make childbirth bearable. The physicians who ease the agonies of cancer sufferers. And, now, we are the men and women who make everyday life easier for thousands of pain patients every day.

When I left the army in 1995, I moved to New York City and joined the anesthesiology staff at Saint Vincent's Hospital. While working at Saint Vincent's, I helped start a pain center in New York City. A "multidisciplinary" pain center has medical doctors, acupuncturists, physical therapists, nutritionists, psychologists, as well as exercise machines and weights, all under one roof.

Several years of working in pain management in different settings led me to develop a four-step program that works to eradicate pain in almost every patient who walks through my door. I hesitate to call it a cure because this program is not an umbrella antidote or a vaccination against all pain. After all, pain still serves a biological purpose for maintaining normal body function. Pain still tells us when something is wrong so that we will fix it. But beyond that, chronic pain need not be endured any longer because we have developed the methods to make pain stop.

These four steps grew out of my on-site research with patients. This is one of the greatest benefits of having many different specialists in one place. I have been able to directly observe what kinds of treatments work, and which ones don't. I am able to immediately see a patient's improvement, the side effects of treatments, and what might cause a recurrence of the pain. I studied the body's natural motion as it emerged from painful states. I monitored patients' stress levels, and sometimes their parallel progress through other diseases such as diabetes or cancer. I studied a patient's lifestyle to find the underlying causes of pain that were not so obvious. I asked patients a lot of questions and listened carefully to their answers. I shared my observations with my colleagues, each adding his or her own expertise to the overall picture. Dr. Bonica's philosophy of pain management was the starting point, but a whole new program evolved from my hands-on daily medical practice as well as from new medications and technologies. The new program was the first of its kind: a unique way of combining treatments and medications that does not allow failure.

One thing was clear from the beginning: using only one remedy or one traditional specialty did not bring a lasting cure. Aspirin, massage, steroid injections, or chiropractors might bring temporary relief, but for a chronic pain patient, none of these by itself is enough to bring permanent relief. Sometimes, when used without overlapping other treatments, they can even make pain worse. Many times, using just two or three methods is not enough. Experience proves that the four stages are necessary to completely break the pain for a lifetime. Here are the four steps of the Painbuster program that are explained in detail in this book.

Step One: Identify the Source of Pain

Finding the reason for pain is the start of treatment.

Listening to patients is a vital element to successful pain management. Doctors must interpret frustrated descriptions of varying degrees of pain, to find clues that will lead to a cure. One person's backache is very distinct from another's, and not just because of individual perception and reaction. Backaches are caused by widely diverse sources and, if the proper source is not targeted, the pain cure will fail. Not only that, but almost every pain ailment will involve different types of pain. For example, a herniated disc might spread pain from the spinal nerve center to a nearby group of back muscles. This person's aching lower back is caused not by nerve pain or muscle pain, but by *both* nerve pain *and* muscle pain. Many doctors are not even aware that both kinds of pain are present in this situation, so they usually prescribe treatment for only one of them. This might mask some of the pain for a while, but it doesn't eliminate the pain. Almost all pain is caused by a combination of pain types, and they will only be completely cured by a combination of treatments.

Step One, identifying the source of pain, begins with a personal interview and a questionnaire that is carefully devised to pinpoint the cause—or rather, the causes—of pain. Although many painful diseases have common symptoms, several individual factors listed on the Painbuster Profile questionnaire, such as a person's employment situation, will affect the treatment. The pain is then classified according to six types of pain: nerve, muscle, bony, visceral, sympathetic, and psychogenic. Most pain syndromes are a combination of at least two of these. For example, a patient who suffers primarily from nerve pain will also acquire muscle pain as a result of the nerve pain.

It is important to indicate that chronic pain can be a symptom of another ailment, and sometimes chronic pain is a disease unto itself. The profile helps us characterize the "syndrome," or the collection of painful symptoms that might indicate a particular disease. By definition, a disease is a malfunctioning of some part or system in the body. Sometimes, the system that is malfunctioning is the body's natural pain control system. Therefore, chronic pain can be a symptom. Several pains might comprise a syndrome. And these pain symptoms or pain syndrome might indicate a disease that is arthritis, tendinitis, or the disease of chronic pain.

Once the cause and the types of pain are determined, treatment can begin. The Painbuster questionnaire is included in this book, starting on page 47, along with instructions on how to use it to help detect the source of your pain.

Step Two: Combat the Pain from Every Angle

No progress toward rehabilitation can be made until the pain is first removed.

Initial treatment varies from person to person, depending on the presence of the six types of pain. The medications that alleviate the pain of sore muscles are a completely different classification from the medications that relieve the nerve pain of sciatica or the bony pain of a broken wrist. Yet a simple muscle ache can compound itself by leaping over to the sympathetic nerves, or triggering neurons to fire pain messages in the brain long after the original injury is healed. Each of these symptoms needs to be treated in different ways. Not all pain relievers work on all pain, a misconception held even by some doctors. I once had a cancer patient who was taking morphine for his tumor pain. Morphine has almost no effect on the bony pain of a growing tumor unless massive amounts are taken, which in this case was not good for the patient. What the patient needed was Motrin, which is superb at stopping bony pain. The patient found it hard to believe that a drug he could buy over the counter was going to be more effective than morphine on his cancer pain, but it was. Sometimes I find that convincing the patient is the most challenging part of a treatment.

Human determination—the simple desire to recover—
is sometimes all it takes to mend a serious pain syndrome.
Scientific studies have proved that 30 percent of all pain
patients will get better, no matter what kind of therapeutic
treatment is used. If patients are told that a pill will relieve
their pain, one-third of them will get well, whether you
give them a sugar pill or actual medication. This is the
"placebo effect." However, it does not work for the other
two-thirds of pain patients. Real medications—either in
pill form or injections, or both—make an enormous difference. And overlapping a variety of medications enables a
doctor and patient to combat the pain from every angle.

A pain specialist monitors all types of pain in every
case, so that each type is appropriately treated. Since most
patients have two or three types of pain together, each is
attacked by one or two methods simultaneously. A prescription pain reliever can be used safely along with other
pain-relieving drugs, such as tricyclic antidepressants,
muscle relaxants, or steroid injections. When they are used
together, each is used in very small doses and with much
greater effect. The traditional usage of these drugs will
not necessarily control pain at all. But the way we use
them—in safe yet nontraditional ways—they become powerful conquerors of pain. This overlapping of medications is
what sets the Painbuster program apart from any other
pain control program. It is the most potent of the four steps,
because it works for almost every patient, and because it
enables the patient to regain normal body motion. We
frequently overlap the medications with another kind
of treatment, such as acupuncture or psychological coun-

seling. These elements often enhance the effectiveness of medications.

If one combination fails to achieve lasting pain relief, we add another medication, or we switch to alternatives in the same medication families. Because we are using very low doses, and because we understand the chemistry of how these drugs work together in the body, we can always find a safe combination that works, no matter what kind of pain you have. Our patients think it is a miracle that we can unlock the right combination to free them from pain. But it is a scientific reality. However, even medications are not the total cure.

Step Three: Commit to Movement Therapy

The goal of eliminating pain with medications is to get you moving again. Pain medication only makes you comfortable enough to exercise, which stops the pain from returning.

Physical therapy is the cure, no matter what disease is causing the pain. Years, months, or even a few days of pain take a heavy toll on the body. Pain affects the movement of the injured area, and it also adds extra stress to the parts that are healthy. When a chronic pain is present, the body naturally recalibrates itself into a revised state of functionality. A person in pain may not even notice that she is walking with a slightly different posture, leaning, limping, or shifting her weight abnormally. The healthy parts pick up the slack, compensating for the pain. In a very short time, the body retains the motion of an injured state as normal motion. Then the healthy parts might start to hurt, too. And the body tries to adjust once again, causing even more unnatural motion and subsequent pain. Little by little, but without fail, pain works in an insidious cycle, dragging a patient into a chronic pain syndrome. Only one thing can stop this degenerative process: physical therapy. A supervised exercise program returns the body to its normal condition prior to the pain—frequently to even better condition than before the injury.

If medication is used without physical therapy, the patient will be pain-free only as long as the medication lasts. We use this to our advantage in Step Three. When the medicated patient enters that pain-free state, he or she begins a series of customized exercises to rebuild body strength. More important than building strength, physical therapy retrains the body to move in a normal way. Returning the body to normal motion gives the pain nowhere to go, except out of the body completely.

Some people object when they hear my program involves the use of medications. But I use them much differently than most doctors have done in the past. I use them to get the patient moving. I endorse the least invasive means that gets rid of a patient's pain *and enables him to exercise.* If acupuncture alone can do it, or meditation, that's great. But most people need a combination of overlapping medications to reach this step. In fact, it is crucial that patients complete Steps One and Two before beginning physical therapy. Some physicians have made the mistake of sending patients out for physical therapy after an injury, without first providing complete pain relief. If the patient is still in pain, physical therapy is counterproductive. It hurts to do it, so the patient does it wrong. Or he might only do the exercises that don't hurt, and skip the ones that cause pain, even though those are usually the most important exercises. Physical therapy is not only crucial to the cure, it is essential that it be performed correctly, and that means when pain is absent.

Some pain patients do not understand how physical therapy can make them well, or they dislike the idea of aerobic classes and lifting weights. Some people believe that surgery might be an easier solution for them than committing to physical therapy would be. Even if you have never exercised in your life, a manageable program can be designed just for you. Movement helps unravel the months or years of contortion and bad "muscle memory." I cannot treat a patient who will not commit to some sort of exercise on which we both agree. There is no point in giving such a patient any medications or other treatment.

Later in the book I will show you some specific exercises that are helpful (and ones that are not helpful), and what kinds of specialists to seek out for help with your commitment to movement therapy.

Step Four:
Customize a Maintenance Program That Works

Once the pain is removed and physical therapy (PT) has reeducated the body, maintenance is the key.

After physical therapy has retrained the body to a normal healthy state, and pain medications are no longer needed, we must take one more step as a precaution against recurrence of the pain. In other words, Step Four ensures that the pain doesn't come back. This step has a multitude of facets, some of which may not be necessary for all patients. These include proper nutrition, stress reduction counseling, regular exercise, emotional support systems, proper posture, and good sleep habits. This step also includes information on what to do for inevitable minor pains, such as muscle soreness after a weekend of raking leaves. Learning how to reduce normal pain correctly, and how to reduce the likelihood of getting these pains, can keep your body from entering another chronic state and starting the cycle all over again.

It is rare that a patient simply returns pain-free to the same life she had before. The transformation of body condition brings a renewed appreciation of good health, and a new awareness of the factors that accompany pain. For example, arthritis patients should know that eating tomatoes or eggplant can aggravate this pain condition in many people, due to the enzymes they contain. Having gone through the first three steps to recover a pain-free lifestyle, the arthritis patient should know to avoid "surprise scallopini" at her celebration dinner.

While some patients have a sense of rebirth after the pain is gone, other people have difficulty adjusting to a life without pain. This is not easy to understand, particularly for the patients who experience it. Maybe pain was the most prevailing aspect of their lives and, without it, they're not sure what to put in its place. In certain cases, the underlying cause of pain might have been a hidden memory, or a foundering relationship that is not yet resolved. Some people have even learned to enjoy life with a little pain ever present in the background. As part of a maintenance program, I support whatever makes the patient comfortable.

One of the most common underlying causes of pain is stress. Most of us are familiar with stress to some degree. It is biological instinct—the "fight or flight" response—for our bodies to tense muscles and adjust blood flow during moments of stress. This is a proven fact. When people speak of "internalizing" a problem, they may not realize what truth they speak. Stress can be particularly taxing on the back muscles, and I believe it is the reason why lower back pain is the dominant syndrome of all my patients. Returning a healthy patient to his old life of stress is a guarantee that I'll be seeing him again before long. To remain pain-free, you must learn new ways to cope with stress, to "externalize" stress in a helpful way and give your poor muscles a break. Pain centers offer group sessions for stress reduction, as well as private counseling, although this is not a program prerequisite as physical therapy is. But when my patients see the scientific evidence connecting stress with chronic pain, they usually want to try at least one group session. They're pleased to discover that stress counseling not only helps control pain, but it improves their lives in other ways.

As with medication therapy, the variable options of pain-free maintenance overlap—the fibromyalgia patient might adjust her diet, take daily walks, and attend regular group-support therapy. If the first three steps serve as a bombing raid against a chronic pain syndrome, this last step acts as a preemptive strike against further assault.

These are Painbuster habits that ensure a pain-free future.

Combining Is Key

Step One correctly identifies the cause of pain. Step Two overlaps the use of different medications to combat the pain from every angle. In Step Three, we show how physical therapy is the goal of using the medications. In Step Four, we discuss overlapping new lifestyles and healthy behavior to keep pain away forever. If any of these steps is taken in isolation, without the other three, this program will not work. For 90 percent of my patients, this program conquers pain completely.

Overlapping treatments of different disciplines prevents the pain from temporarily shifting to another part of your body while the original location gets the medical attention. Most pain sufferers and even their doctors start with solitary medications such as Tylenol or Motrin and, after their effects wear off (as all drugs do, in time), they might step up to Tylenol with codeine. Meanwhile, the pain might have spread from a nerve to a nearby muscle, changing its original nature into something else. The new type of pain may very well not respond to Tylenol at all. So now, after only a couple of weeks, you might have two different pains reverberating back and forth, developing into a wider and more complicated syndrome that will eventually embed the pain messages into your system.

The simultaneous assaults of the Painbuster program leave the pain nowhere to go. Because we overlap two or three medications with a rotating exercise program, and massage or acupuncture or stress therapy, we can annihilate the most tenacious pain, even pain that has lived in your body for a long time.

A few years ago, a new patient arrived in my office at the pain center. Megan B. was a striking woman in her forties, with beautiful dark hair and eyes. She was an officer at a bank during the week and raced a forty-foot sailboat with her husband on weekends. A couple of years earlier, Megan had wrenched her back the wrong way while pulling up the mainsail. After several weeks of taking Tylenol, her muscle spasm did not go away, so she went to an orthopedist. The doctor prescribed Flexeril, a muscle relaxant, and advised her to rest. The Flexeril had little effect, so Megan followed a friend's advice and went to see a chiropractor. The chiropractor treatment made her feel better. Although she refrained from arduous exercise— even from sailing—the pain soon returned, only this time the pain was different. It was shooting around from her back to her rib cage.

Frustrated by the go-around of medical treatments, Megan sought out a new orthopedist. This doctor gave her Xanax to calm her anxiety and to help her relax. Megan then joined a meditation class, whose instructor told her that she probably had fibromyalgia, a chronic pain syndrome, and she recommended a new diet and herbal supplements.

Two years later, Megan's pain was as bad as ever. She resolved to try psychological counseling and, along the way, she found the number for my pain center in the phone book. She called for an appointment, without the usual referral from another doctor, which is how many patients find me. Determined to find a cure, Megan had found me on her own.

She walked slightly sideways into my office and pulled out a large green cushion from under her arm. She sat down on it gingerly at the edge of an office chair. As she told me the history of her injury and its many treatments, tears came to her eyes from time to time. At the end of her story, she took a deep breath.

"I know it's probably all in my head," she told me, her shoulders tensing in frustration. "If only I could control my mind a little better, the pain would go away. But when I try it, I think it hurts even more. I really hate to be a complainer, but sometimes I just want to scream!"

I examined Megan's Painbuster Profile questionnaire and asked a few more questions. After talking for a few minutes, I began to see that she had a classic chronic pain syndrome—muscle spasm, compounded by intercostal neuritis (the nerve pain in her rib cage), which was indeed building toward a case of fibromyalgia. Megan seemed uneasy about getting a steroid injection, which I had recommended for immediate relief. Instead, I prescribed the nonsteroidal anti-inflammatory Motrin in conjunction with Zoloft, a tricyclic antidepressant. I have found a number of medications not commonly used to treat pain, such as Zoloft, that have a powerful effect on pain. Zoloft works not on the perception of pain—which people frequently assume—but it actually repairs the damaged nerve pathways carrying repetitive pain messages to the brain. In Megan's case, Motrin and Zoloft would work together to calm the irritated muscle and the overactive nerve pain.

This would take a week or so to achieve the effects of an injection, but it made her more comfortable. I instructed Megan to return in a week to begin physical therapy, if she felt well enough to try it.

One week later, all of Megan's pain was gone, and she began a new exercise routine at my pain center, three times a week. Within a month, she stopped taking the Motrin and joined a weekly group for stress therapy. After twelve weeks of physical therapy, I took her off the Zoloft. Step by careful step, Megan's pain disappeared for good. In the year since she limped into my office, her pain has not resurfaced. Her body strength returned to normal, and she is sailing regularly with her husband again. She recently started a less stressful job and, with the renewed vitality of someone who discovered a "fountain of youth," she and her husband are planning to adopt a baby.

It is not uncommon to find prolonged undertreatment for chronic pain. Studies have shown that the least treated pain patients are women (who have a higher tolerance of pain than men do), racial and ethnic minorities, children, the elderly, those who receive workers' compensation, and those previously disabled by ailments such as blindness or polio.

Jim D., a thirty-two-year-old stonemason, was a patient who came to see me four years ago with a herniated disc. The pain in his lower back was horrible, and it was shooting down his legs. Sometimes he felt as if his knees would buckle. He was unable to work or to do much of anything for that matter. He spent a lot of time lying on the floor. In fact, his wife had driven him to my office while he lay in the back of a van. In Jim's case, the disc was pressing against the nerve roots in his lower spine. Sensing this pain, his back muscles had entered a protective mode by contracting themselves into a spasmodic state. Jim's pain made him restless, so he didn't reach REM ("rapid eye movement") sleep. This meant his overtaxed back muscles never got a chance to relax. Myofascial pain is from spasms of the skeletal muscles, and muscles only relax completely when the body is in REM sleep. REM sleep is the stage at the end of a sleep cycle that requires three to four hours of uninterrupted sleep. Everyone knows how it feels to experience a restless night. Imagine having restless nights for weeks on end! This can certainly exacerbate the original pain syndrome.

The first day I saw Jim, I gave him an epidural steroid injection, and he was able to walk out the door with an amazed smile of relief. I also prescribed Elavil, a tricyclic antidepressant. The Elavil was to be taken at night, since it also has a slight sedative effect, and this would help him get enough sleep to reach that important REM stage, enabling the back muscles to get some rest, too.

I asked Jim to return in three days. When I saw him again, he felt slight residual pain in his lower back, so I gave him another injection, followed by a third injection a week later. By then, the pain was gone from both his back and his legs. He couldn't believe it. We started him on a physical therapy program, and trained him on proper body mechanics to use when he was back on the job. It is possible to do heavy lifting without damaging your back and, once Jim understood these dynamics, I knew he would remember them for a lifetime. People who emerge from a state of pain are some of the most motivated people I know. After three months on the Painbuster program, armed with a new exercise routine to do at home, Jim went back to work. His insurance company later telephoned to thank me for not recommending surgery to cure Jim's back injury! My cure had saved them a lot of money.

There are cases where our initial treatment may fall short of achieving complete pain relief. If we discover that the tricyclic antidepressant is not having the desired effect on a patient's nerve pain, we may try another kind of medication instead. We might add an injection of local anesthetic into a nerve plexus. Or we might move on to a new medication combination, such as a mild muscle relaxant with a tricyclic antidepressant. Sometimes the initial medication combination is terrific for a few weeks, then begins to wear off. We might then rotate medications, to attack the pain from a new angle. When you overlap multiple combinations, in small, safe doses, the pain has no chance of surviving.

In most cases, I can achieve better pain relief without surgery. After all, surgery itself is an added painful procedure, and I always prefer treatments that are the least invasive, and the least painful. In some cases—and only a select few—after rotating through a number of techniques and medications, it becomes apparent that the pain will only be eliminated through an advanced technique, such as freezing a small nerve, or with some kind of surgical procedure. I use these methods as a last resort because they are irreversible. Unlike the four-step program, if the advanced procedure or surgery does not relieve the pain, there is no recourse for the damaged nerve or surgical scarring. I have a lot of experience performing advanced procedures that

are effective. And I have also observed patients who choose
to have surgeries that didn't have a chance of eliminating
their pain. My goal is to help the patient make the most
informed decision possible, and only after exhausting all
the noninvasive options. As I said earlier, almost all of my
pain patients are cured without surgery—and my patients
have been in chronic pain for a very long time. But sometimes even I can see the benefits of surgery in certain cases,
and they are reviewed in chapter 8.

Many other doctors work in conjunction with me to
help patients control pain. An endocrinologist may refer his
diabetic patient to me, so I can treat the burning pain in his
patient's hands and feet. That doctor continues to treat the
patient's diabetes; I treat his pain. An oncologist may ask
me to consult with a cancer patient and help resolve the
pain of her tumor. I don't treat cancer, but I do understand
why tumors cause pain, and how the pain can be stopped
without impeding her normal alertness and activity. Of
course, most of my patients don't have diabetes or cancer.
They have chronic pain diseases such as arthritis, herniated
disc, or complex regional pain syndrome. Many times, the
only doctor they need is a pain-management specialist.

Without access to a pain-management specialist, the
best primary health provider is the pain patient herself,
assisted by an internist or general practitioner. Educated
pain patients who understand what's happened to their
own bodies, and how and why they hurt, can understand
what treatment will work for them. Pain remedies make
sense when you are aware of them, and when you understand the causes and the changing nature of pain. *Painbuster* provides an arsenal of treatment techniques in the

four steps that really work to eliminate chronic pain, and explains how you can use them with your doctor. This book tells you what specific treatments are available, which ones are most effective for your specific ailment, and how you can find them.

Each of the four steps in the Painbuster program is explained in its own chapter. For special pain syndromes, such as those experienced by cancer sufferers or people with terminal illnesses, there are additional sections. This book also contains an A-to-Z glossary of pain syndromes and symptoms, listing the most effective overlapping treatment methods for each one. You will discover every option available, how each one works and, just as importantly, which ones don't work.

Painbuster encompasses the techniques I have refined in my lifelong career as a pain-management specialist. In order for you to fully benefit from this program, you should share the information in this book with your doctor or seek out a pain specialist from the resource directory provided in chapter 10. Once you are familiar with the Painbuster program, you and your doctor can discuss the specific options described here. Doctors will agree that these treatment suggestions are safe, and many of them should be able to implement the program in partnership with you.

Removing the mystery and frustration from the traditional treatment of chronic pain—for both patient and doctor—is an important element to the success of pain management. You are now on your way to good health. I will guide you through the rest of the journey toward freedom from pain.

CHAPTER 2

Why It Hurts

Step One: Identify the Cause of the Pain

David S. is a fifty-nine-year-old hospital administrator who came to see me with tendinitis, the classic ailment known as "tennis elbow." He had been taking Motrin for several weeks, while resting his elbow, and had recently even tried acupuncture to ease the pain. After three months, he was restless. He was eager to play tennis again, but his arm still hurt. He came to see me about a cortisone injection for his sore arm.

It took very little time for me to observe that David did not have tendinitis. His elbow pain caused radiating shivers up his arm and throughout his body. For a few moments, I considered whether David might have a hairline fracture. But the shooting pain down his arm was more symptomatic of cervical radiculopathy. This nerve ailment is essentially sciatica of the neck. Instead of sciatica of the lower back, which sends nerve pain down someone's leg, this sciatica-like pain was in David's neck area, sending lancing pains down his arm. We gave David an epidural steroid injection in his neck, near the seventh cervical vertebra, and he was fine. He never even needed another injection. He started playing tennis again within a week. David could have had the remedy for his sore elbow months earlier, but a mistaken diagnosis diverted him from the true cure to one that had no effect at all.

The first step in the Painbuster program is to identify the source of pain. Studies show that half of all pain patients are not properly diagnosed in the first place. This might lead to needless months of suffering and frustration that can, in turn, compound a simple injury into a chronic pain syndrome. Pain is subjective. It cannot be clinically measured and each individual has her own tolerance level, a unique pain experience that depends on variables such as overall health and the nature of the injury. But we have learned how to ask the proper questions that will give us informative answers. At my pain center, I begin with a personal interview as well as a written questionnaire. I immediately use this information to help classify the types of pain involved.

The Six Types of Pain

All the different pain syndromes that exist in the world can be broken down into just six components. They are:

- nerve pain, which occurs when a large nerve or group of small nerves has been damaged;

- visceral pain, the evasive aches from the gut associated with internal organs;
- myofascial pain, which consists of aches or swelling of muscle and tissue;
- bony pain, such as arthritis, which usually occurs in the joints;
- sympathetic pain, which occurs when the sympathetic nerves have started sending pain messages out of control; and
- psychogenic pain, which is real pain from no physiological cause.

In almost every case, a person's pain syndrome involves two or three types of pain, a combination that must be determined before effective treatment can begin. Then, by treating each part individually, we topple the entire pain syndrome, no matter how long it's been there, or how severe it is.

A patient with a herniated disc and a shooting pain down her leg, for example, will usually also have muscle spasms in her back as a result of this pain condition. We have to treat the spasmodic pain—which is myofascial— in addition to her nerve pain. These require two very different healing methods. Only after taking the time and effort to distinguish these elements can we begin the right cure.

A pain sufferer can understand a great deal about his syndrome if he understands the variety of pain types. Most people know that a burn injury hurts differently than a twisted knee, but they don't usually know why. On the following pages are the distinctions that pain-management specialists, as well as other doctors, use to clarify the different ways that you hurt and why.

NERVE PAIN

Sensory nerves are the branches that lead from the spinal cord to every part of the body, to the internal organs, and to the fingertips. The nerves absorb information through receptors, such as a pain signal, and transmit this information to the brain. There are two different kinds of nerve, or neuropathic, pain: large nerve pain and small nerve pain. Nerves with large diameters feel sharp pains that shoot up and down the entire nerve—like the shooting leg pains of sciatica. The large nerve injury of sciatica is usually at the lumbar area of the lower spine, but the nerve radiates pain throughout the entire length of the area it serves, in this case, the leg. People describe this pain as being as sharp as a lightning bolt. Another example of large nerve pain is hitting one's "funny bone." This is not a bone, but actually the ulnar nerve as it passes through the elbow. You feel the pain shoot down your whole arm and out your fingers. Large nerve pain can occur at any point along the large nerve, but it usually hurts more when the injury is at the nerve's starting area, where it is the largest in diameter. If you hurt the sciatic nerve farther down your leg, it will hurt less because it has less distance to shoot through.

Small nerve pain has less distinct borders. Instead of being sharp-shooting, the pain is more diffuse: a burning, itching pain that many patients find hard to describe. One

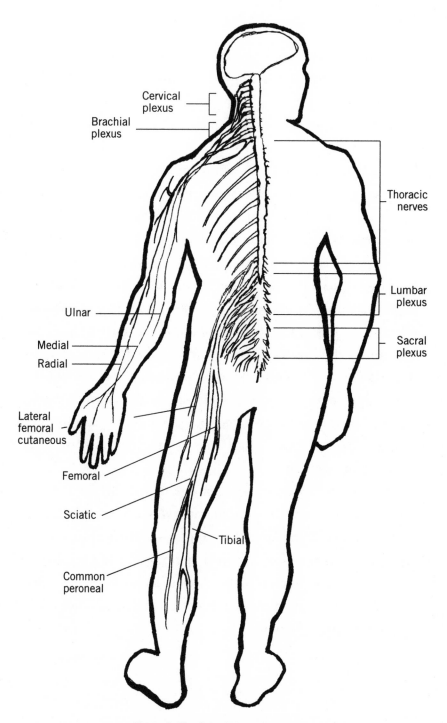

Figure 1: The Spinal Nervous System
The various nerves interconnect at plexuses, as shown.

example of small nerve pain is a sunburn. Diabetics sometimes experience a burning sensation in their hands and
feet. We call this "stocking-glove" distribution of pain,
because the pain strikes where one would wear socks and
gloves—in other words, in and near the hands and feet.
This pain syndrome is known as diabetic polyneuropathy
and is caused by damage across a whole group of small
nerve endings. Because the damage occurs over a fairly
widespread area, the pain also feels spread out and difficult to pinpoint.

Small nerve pain can also be a side effect of radiation
therapy, caused by exposure to a toxin, or from a metabolic
event that has injured a broad area of nerves, such as
ischemia, which is the decreased blood flow to the extremities. Ischemia is common among older people. Ischemia
can trigger nerve impulses to the brain that something is
"amiss" in the hands and feet, but instead of a tingling or
"funny" feeling, the small nerves might transmit this
information as pain.

The most common large nerve pain syndromes include
sciatica (also known as lumbar radiculopathy), toothaches,
and herniated discs. Small nerve pains include skin burns,
shingles (herpes zoster), diabetic pain, and the peripheral
neuropathy frequently associated with alcoholism. You
should consult a pain-management specialist or a neurologist for this type of pain.

VISCERAL PAIN

Each organ in the abdomen has a membrane, or balloon-like capsule, that surrounds it. Visceral pain comes from a stretch or irritation of any of these hollow viscous areas in the body, such as the capsules that hold the heart and liver. It might also be from the bowels, the kidneys, or the lining of the lungs. When one of these organs swells, perhaps due to an injury or other inflammation, the organ pushes against the capsule surrounding it. The body senses this pain, but it can't sense the exact location. It is a widespread gripping, deep ache, similar to a gas pain. When visceral pain occurs, it is not obvious what is causing it, nor what can be done to alleviate it.

If a fingertip is injured, it is fairly easy to pinpoint the source of pain. But in the visceral "gut" area, there are a lot of pain receptors that feed into a single nerve pathway, so it's more difficult to determine which receptor is feeling the pain. Because of this range of pain receptors, we can be fooled by which one is the culprit. The body is indicating that something is wrong, but we cannot tell where the exact source is.

A classic example of how visceral pain can be deceptive is when a patient has had laparoscopic surgery, perhaps for removal of the gallbladder. In this surgery a fiberoptic instrument is inserted through a small incision in the abdominal wall, and carbon dioxide is used to inflate the abdomen during surgery. Aleesha G. had this operation, and residual pain remained not only in her abdomen, but in her shoulders and back. There was gas left over in her abdominal cavity from the procedure, which had irritated the area, including the nerves from her lower spine to her upper back.

This is probably the most difficult type of pain to control, because the pain is evasive and the area encompasses so many different organs. The best pain remedy in these cases is to cure the underlying ailment. The abdomen encompasses organs treated by many different specialists (the bowel, the liver, the appendix, the uterus, and so on) and I work with many of them to control a patient's visceral pain. Visceral pain might include that of peptic ulcer, irritable bowel syndrome, endometriosis, reflux esophagitis, or pleuritis.

MYOFASCIAL PAIN

Myofascial (or tissue) pain includes muscle spasm, swelling of tissue, and broken or injured bones. It is a very broad category, mostly because human tissue is more exposed than any other part of the body. Tissue includes the skin, the muscles, and bone. There are many receptors throughout this group, and trauma to any one of them signals danger to the entire body. This family also has a large number of reflex reactions: a painful stimulus will cause all nearby muscles or tissue to tense and protect the area, perhaps causing a spasm around the original injury. As time passes, the original injury will usually heal itself, but the secondary spasm might linger and turn into a separate pain syndrome all its own.

Lower back injury, such as a herniated disc, almost

always involves myofascial pain. A muscle spasm occurs when the muscle is stretched or overworked, causing it to contract into a protective mode. A "charley horse" pain and the pain from lifting a heavy suitcase out of a car trunk are acute muscle spasms you might readily recognize. The charley horse is actually a large group of muscles contracting in unison. The back spasm is more localized, maybe involving just one or two small muscles but, in most instances, it can be even more painful than a charley horse.

Three things happen during a muscle spasm. First, the spasm activity releases lactic acid into the immediate area. Lactic acid is a natural by-product of any work done by any muscle. When a muscle spasms, it is more or less working overtime, involuntarily. As the muscle works and works and works through a spasm, it is releasing as much lactic acid as if it were running in a marathon. If you were really running a marathon, the increased blood flow would carry this lactic acid away to your liver, where it is broken down and eventually excreted. If you are having a spasm and not running a marathon, however, this extra lactic acid is being produced in the local area, but there is no increased blood flow to carry it away quickly enough. Because of the buildup of lactic acid, the muscle has no chance to relax and recover—it behaves as though it still has a lot of lactic acid to eliminate. As far as your muscles are concerned, you are only halfway through your marathon, with several miles more to go. But you know you are gripped by a muscle spasm, and not running anywhere. The lactic acid makes the affected muscles very sore. The lactic acid buildup also irritates the surrounding muscles, and will most likely cause them to spasm, too. This new spasm continues until all the muscles stop, or until the lactic acid dissipates.

The second thing that happens during a muscle spasm is that other muscles around the injured area work harder to maintain balance, compensating for the muscles that are locked in a spasm. Almost every muscle in the body has a corresponding "contralateral" muscle that performs its exact opposite task. Picture your lower back: the muscles on each side of your spine work against each other to keep your spine centered and straight. These muscles are almost mirror images of one another. During a spasm, one side is pulled too hard, forcing you to lean over to one side. But the body tries to compensate by using the muscles on the opposite side to counteract the spasm's pull and keep your spine straight. This eventually causes fatigue to the overworked healthy muscle and it will start to spasm, too, unless it is treated as well. It becomes easy to see how spasms can radiate much farther from the original injury.

The third thing that happens during a spasm is that the muscle develops a new "memory" of the spasmodic position. Golf pros frequently use the term *muscle memory* to help golfers play better. In golf terms, the muscle's memory of your swinging motion can help you consistently hit long drives from the tee. But for a pain patient, muscle memory is not a good thing to have. For muscles not only retain a memory of motion, they retain a memory of inertia, too. Muscles have a memory of their normal resting state. When not in use, each muscle returns to this state again and again, as they await commands from your nervous system for a new task. Once a muscle has been locked in a spasm, it begins to remember this as its normal state. When not in action, the muscle returns to this state over and over again. But this painfully locked spasm is not, of course, its normal state.

Dave C. is a thirty-nine-year-old housepainter who also happens to play a lot of golf. After a fall from a ladder, he injured a ligament in his left instep. It seemed like a minor foot injury, and it should have been. Dave was so busy at work that his foot remained untreated for several weeks, during which time he unconsciously perfected a limp—a new muscle memory—that compensated for his injured foot and enabled him to keep up his hectic schedule. After a while, Dave's ligament healed but, by then, the over-taxed, spasming muscles in his right foot were killing him. An orthopedist provided Dave with an orthotic device to put in his right shoe, which would take some of the weight off his aching contralateral muscles.

An orthotic is something I almost never recommend because all it does is help your foot learn an unnatural muscle memory. Orthotics can be helpful for certain people who were born with naturally poor alignment, but they are not usually helpful in treating injuries. Dave's new orthotic started changing the gait on his left foot—the same foot that suffered the ligament injury in the first place. With the added stress of unnatural muscle memo-ries in both feet, the tender ligament was easily damaged again, and suddenly Dave had a whole symphony of pain types in both feet. He not only needed medication, but also intensive short-term retraining on how to walk correctly. I prescribed a nonsteroidal anti-inflammatory, a muscle relaxant, and replaced his orthotic device with a specific exercise routine. Within a month, he was fine.

Another kind of patient who is prone to this type of pain is a frequent traveler or someone who often carries heavy bags. This person might be a sales representative, carrying a laptop on one shoulder and dragging a brief-case with the other hand, completely out of balance and frequently reinjuring the same shoulder with every trip, over and over again. Treatment must include retraining the muscle to its normal resting state instead of its spasmodic resting state. Once the memory has established itself, it becomes more difficult to treat it and retrain the muscle. And the longer a muscle pain remains in the body, the harder it is to cure. The spasm has an insidious effect on posture, motion, and normal functions of the afflicted area.

Muscle spasm is the most common secondary pain, which means it is the one most likely to accompany any other primary pain—nerve pain, visceral pain, and even another muscle pain—in the area that hurts. The nearby muscle is instinctively trying to protect the injured area. If you herniate a disc in your lower back, the radicular nerve pain shoots down your leg. Not only does the large nerve pain cause the lower back muscles to spasm, but it will cause you to limp, or to ever-so-slightly change your balance as you walk. This side effect causes different, nearby muscles in your lower back to spasm, too. The radicular nerve pain might get resolved with appropriate treatment but, frequently, doctors don't treat that additional back spasm because they're not aware of the distinction. So the pain continues. And the limping perpetuates the pain because the patient hasn't been retrained to walk properly.

Almost all myofascial pain syndromes are accompanied by stress, which further exacerbates pain. In fact, stress is a greater factor in myofascial pain than with any other kind of pain. People generally "feel" stress in their upper or lower back muscles. Most medical researchers believe that the stress hormones in humans—norepinephrine and epinephrine—are also mediators of pain. If your muscle is on the verge of a spasm and a lot of stress hormones are moving around, that spasm won't be long in coming. A muscle spasm that turns into chronic myofascial pain frequently evolves into fibromyalgia, a serious pain disease. If all the symptoms that comprise myofascial pain syndromes are not quickly resolved, they can stick around for years.

Muscle spasms in the back are most often caused by twisting and lifting at the same time, like standing up from a chair the wrong way, or lifting a heavy carton off a truck. They are also commonly caused by reaching out and carrying something with your arms extended, such as lifting a child from a car seat or a suitcase from the trunk. Injuries are also common at health clubs that promote weight lifting, and with people who overdo it on weekend yard work and exercise. An orthopedist understands how to alleviate muscle pain. Remember, however, that this type of pain is usually intertwined with another type, one that an orthopedist might not immediately recognize. In most cases of myofascial pain, I recommend a pain-management specialist so that the syndrome does not last too long and become more difficult to resolve.

BONY PAIN

Bone pain is a very distinct and easily identified pain. The bones in the body are the support structure for all its motion. There are fibers that coat the bone and the surrounding tissue that clings tightly to the bone, known as periosteum. If there is any disruption of this tissue covering the bone, such as a broken leg, extreme pain is caused by the damaged periosteum. A broken bone has lost its structural integrity and it hurts when it is moved. You cannot walk on a broken leg.

Another cause of bony pain is when the periosteum is stretched instead of broken, as with the growth of metastatic lesions in a cancer patient. Even though the cancer might be primarily rooted in an organ, cancer cells sometimes travel to other parts of the body. If the cells attach to a bone, a lesion might grow that takes up space, enlarging the bone itself. This will stretch the periosteum, causing pain. Certain cancers, like prostate or cervical cancer, have a tendency to metastasize to a bone and cause tumors to grow in the bone. Alternatively, a metastatic lesion might erode the bone and irritate the periosteum by weakening it, making all movement painful. Sometimes this type of lesion will weaken the bone to the point of breaking it, in what is called a pathological fracture. What began as a slow-growing pain then becomes the acute pain of a broken bone.

Pain from the bone, and from the periosteum, is caused by the release of the prostaglandin known as substance P. Prostaglandins are fatty acids that normally protect certain parts of the body, such as the lining of the stomach. Sub-

stance P, however, is a neurotransmitter of pain. It activates
the sensory nervous system to send pain messages to the
brain. Substance P also causes inflammation (the medical
term for swelling), which adds another irritation to what
started out as simple bony pain. One of the best defenses
against substance P is a nonsteroidal anti-inflammatory,
such as Motrin or Aleve. An orthopedist can treat this,
as long as she is aware of the presence of substance P, in
addition to the injured periosteum. Bony pain syndromes
include not only broken bones and dislocations, but arthritis, tumors, injured vertebrae, and osteoporosis.

SYMPATHETIC PAIN

Sympathetic pain gets its name from the sympathetic
nervous system, which consists of nerves located throughout the body. While sensory nerves are responsible for conscious motion and response to stimulus such as hot and
cold, sympathetic nerves control breathing, blood pressure,
and heartbeat. These activities are not under conscious
control and are sometimes affected by emotions like fear or
anger.

One of the functions of the sympathetic nerves is to
regulate blood flow to all parts of the body. These nerves
can change blood flow in an instant, with the reflex movement called the "fight or flight" response. If a muscle is
going to be needed to defend the body, say in the legs so
they might run away from danger, the sympathetic nervous
system senses the emotional stress. The sympathetic nerves
rush blood to that part of the body, the legs, as they slow

blood flow to other areas that need it less, such as the digestive area. Studies show that even anticipation of pain can trigger the area in the brain that controls the sympathetic nervous system. Simple anxiety about the dentist's drill can trigger the brain unconsciously, building anticipation until the actual pain response is more intense than it would have been without the anxiety. Fear of pain can be worse than pain itself, because it adds sympathetic pain to the mixture.

Sympathetic nerves are very small and fragile, with little protection. They can be injured by the slightest trauma. Dr. Silas Weir Mitchell first described sympathetic pain during the American Civil War, when so many advances in pain management were discovered. Among thousands of patients with bullet wounds and amputations, Weir Mitchell observed a patient whose pain was different. He noticed that the patient's gunshot wound had not caused any sensory nerve damage, yet his pain was wildly out of proportion. The original injury was prompting neurons to "recruit" the sympathetic nerve cells to respond as if they, too, were receiving pain signals. The damage to his sympathetic nerve was sending pain messages to the sensory nerve, which echoed back and forth into a vicious cycle that enhanced the pain enormously. It's like having crossed telephone wires, when you suddenly join someone else's conversation and you can't disconnect from them. Damage to a sensory nerve causes nerve pain. Damage to a sympathetic nerve causes sympathetic pain. Today, we see many conditions that cause sympathetic pain from minor surgical procedures at extremities like the foot or hand, or a sprained ankle when someone wears a tight boot, or in a patient who has to wear a cast after surgery.

The symptoms of sympathetic pain are called allodynia, which is another name for a painful response to a nonpainful stimulus. We test for this with a light touch over an area. The patient often feels intense pain and doesn't want anything touching that sensitive spot, not even a piece of clothing. When we see this kind of response, we know the sympathetic nervous system is in overdrive. Other symptoms include edema, or swelling, in the area. Increase in blood flow makes the area hot and swollen. The greatest challenge to sympathetic pain is recognizing it quickly enough and treating it immediately, so the pain does not settle in for a long time. We eradicate sympathetic pain with nerve block injections into various points along the sympathetic nerve system.

Sympathetic pain syndromes include reflex sympathetic dystrophy (now called complex regional pain syndrome, Type II). This is where there is no apparent damage, yet sympathetic nerves have somehow connected to sensory nerves to transmit pain messages to the brain. Another such syndrome is causalgia (or complex regional pain syndrome, Type I), where there is actual damage to a nerve. Treatment is always targeted at breaking the linkage of the crossed wires, which is what nerve block injections can do. Most neurologists are very knowledgeable about treating this type of pain.

PSYCHOGENIC PAIN

This last pain type is probably the most difficult to describe. Psychogenic pain is the state where there is no apparent physiological cause for the pain. Although there may be no anatomical reason to explain it, this does not mean the pain doesn't exist. In fact, psychogenic pain is very real, and it can be incapacitating.

Some doctors mistake this pain as the symptom of a malingering patient who wants to feign a pain syndrome for other reasons. Without a diagnostic test for pain, it is possible for someone to fake it from time to time. New magnetic resonance imaging (MRI) technology is beginning to offer hope that pain will more easily be identified in brain scans, because psychogenic pain is very real. Unlike the malingerer, a patient with psychogenic pain has real pain, and no control over it. It is as severe as the pain from a broken bone, and it needs to be treated just as seriously. Many pain syndromes are accompanied by some degree of psychogenic pain. It can surface even after the other pain symptoms are healed. If we have treated every known physical source of pain correctly, the pain should not return. If the pain does return, that part of it may be the psychogenic remnants of the original complaint.

The key to resolving psychogenic pain is to find out why the patient has it—what is stopping the patient from getting better. Psychogenic pain is rarely generated by the area of the original injury. Much of it is real pain caused by the shift in a patient's attitude, such as someone who is filled with despair that he will never be healed. Psychogenic pain may strike someone who falls into the depression that inevitably accompanies chronic pain. Psychogenic pain may not have any connection to the original pain ailment, but that's exactly where it might manifest itself. If psychogenic pain is not addressed separately, it can develop into a chronic pain syndrome.

We treat this pain with the same remedies that are used for the other five pain types, depending on which one the psychogenic pain presents. I have found that working with psychologists to help change a patient's attitude can be very helpful for this pain. And many psychologists work together with doctors like me on such cases. I attack the pain from the physical side, and the counseling helps attack it from the emotional side. We team up to combat the pain from all directions, until it is vanquished.

Most other doctors are not experienced in successfully treating psychogenic pain. In fact, most doctors are familiar with treating only two or three of these six types of pain. A pain-management specialist is familiar with all of the pain types, and how they form combinations. *Painbuster* explains how they work together, and how they can be unraveled and cast away.

The Painbuster Profile

The key to successfully identifying which elements are involved in a patient's pain syndrome is this: Ask the right questions, and you will get the answers you need. When I read the patient's Painbuster Profile, I can find clues that indicate the true source of pain. Actually the true *sources* of pain because, as we now know, there is usually more than one condition causing your pain. For example, a patient's sleep habits reveal a lot about a particular syndrome. If the patient has a condition that includes a muscle spasm—as so many pain syndromes do—it is vital to her recovery that the patient get at least four hours of uninterrupted sleep each night, so that her muscles can relax completely in REM sleep. If the pain awakens my patient every two or three hours, she is never getting to REM sleep. Her body is never reaching muscle relaxation either. This is one example of a clue that can be found in a profile.

It is important to find out what makes pain worse, and what makes it feel better. Someone with a shoulder pain that occurs only when he is using the computer keyboard probably needs better ergonomics at his desk to achieve a lasting cure. Lifestyle questions are also important. People who work out at the gym will often get certain kinds of muscle pain. Exercise—even without obvious stress or injury—can cause muscle pain. Adding a new exercise or changing an exercise routine can cause a different kind of pain. People who work out feel they are being very attentive to their health and are naturally confused when they experience pain instead.

In my practice, after I read the Painbuster Profile and review it with a patient, I look for clues—the symptoms—to link up with a syndrome. I can immediately sort the symptoms into the six basic categories, which help pinpoint the causes of the pain. This profile is frequently accompanied by visual references, such as an X ray or MRI. Here is a review of the most common tests that might show the nature of a structural problem causing your pain.

DIAGNOSTIC TESTS

X ray: This is the best test for looking at bones to determine fractures or displacement of bone structures. The X-ray image does not show soft tissue injuries, however, so something like a disc herniation would require an MRI.

MRI (magnetic resonance imaging): This is probably the most common test used in a pain-management practice. An MRI uses the fluctuations of magnetic waves through the body to produce an image that shows soft tissues rather than bones. This test involves lying on a narrow bed that slides into what is, essentially, a giant magnet. This is why anyone who has metal in her body—a pacemaker, for instance, or nontitanium artificial joints—cannot have an MRI. For some, lying in a narrow space for fifteen minutes is very uncomfortable and claustrophobic. Fortunately, there are now "open" MRI machines that provide a little more space, although the closed MRI is preferred for a sharper picture. The MRI is an excellent test for seeing herniated discs and pressure on nerve roots, among other soft tissue ailments.

CAT (computerized axial tomography) scan: Sometimes also known simply as a CT, this imaging technique is older than the MRI, but it still has useful applications. The CAT scan is made from multiple X-ray images that are reassembled to form a two-dimensional perspective. This is a good test for problems involving bones or soft tissue.

EMG (electromyographic) biofeedback: This is what we call a "provocative" test, to measure nerve damage. The

EMG measures the speed of electrical currents along nerve pathways. If the conduction of electricity is slower than what is considered normal, or if it is different on one side of the body than the other, then we would consider that there's damage along the nerve. This is a good test for observing the changes of nerve damage over time, to document healing. It is also helpful in pinpointing the exact area of damage along a nerve path.

The EMG procedure requires the insertion of several needles into the muscles along the nerve path, and the test takes about thirty or forty minutes. It is not the most comfortable test for a patient, but it is very helpful in pinpointing the source of pain.

Bone scan: This uses the introduction of a radioactive "dye" to show increased blood flow to a bone, when compared to the patient's unaffected bones. This is a safe test, and the increase of blood flow might confirm the diagnosis of an infection, metastatic lesion, acute fracture, or the early stages of complex regional pain syndrome (what was once called reflex sympathetic dystrophy). The bone scan is a simple injection of a very safe compound into the appropriate vein.

These tests are very helpful in our diagnosis, but I find the following questionnaire just as enlightening. I'll explain each part in detail after you review all of them.

Painbuster Profile
PATIENT QUESTIONNAIRE

A. Today's Date:_____/_____/_____

Your information:

Last Name:_____First:_____Middle:_____

Date of Birth:_____/_____/_____ Age:_____SS#:_____

Street:_____City:_____State:_____ Zip Code:_____

Home Phone: (___)_____Work Phone: (___)_____

Emergency Contact:

Name:_____

Street:_____City:_____State:_____ Zip Code:_____

Home Phone: (___)_____ Work Phone: (___)_____

Referring Physician:

Name:_____Specialty:_____

Street:_____ City:_____ State:_____ Zip Code:_____

Phone: (___)_____Fax: (___)_____

Primary Care Physician (PCP):

Name:_____

Street:_____City:_____ State:_____ Zip Code:_____

Phone: (___)_____Fax: (___)_____

Pharmacy:

Name:_____

Street:_____City:_____ State:_____ Zip Code:_____

Phone: (___)_____

We can share information with your

Spouse:_____ significant other: _____ parent: _____children: _____ PCP:_____

Signature:_____

Marital status:_____ Number of children:_____

With whom do you live? _____

Do you practice any religion or have a personal faith system that helps you to cope with the pain?

_____

B. Please describe your pain complaint and how it started:

When did you first experience your pain, and how has it changed since that time?

Please indicate on the following what makes the pain better, worse, or has no effect:

___ Heat	___ Cold	___ Humidity
___ Sitting	___ Standing	___ Lying Down
___ Coughing	___ Fatigue	___ Vibrations
___ Noise	___ Anxiety/Emotions	___ Massage
___ Alcohol	___ Caffeine	___ Body position
___ Sneezing	___ Stairs	___ Bowel movements

Is your pain worse with any particular activities?

0	1	2	3	4	5	6	7	8	9	10
no pain		mild	discomforting			distressing		horrible		excruciating

Using this pain scale, please describe your pain:
- at its worst? _____
- at its least? _____
- right now? _____
- most of the time? _____

Circle any of the following that you currently use:

Cane	Wheelchair	Crutches	Brace
Scooter	Walker	Prosthesis	Collar

Please circle any treatments you have undergone for your pain problem. Place a (+) next to those that were effective and a (-) next to those that were not:

Acupuncture	Hypnosis	TENS (Transartaneous Electrical
Bed rest	Massage	Nerve Stimulation)
Biofeedback	Nerve blocks	Traction
Chiropractor	Physical therapy	Trigger point injections
Epidural steroid injections	Psychotherapy	Ultrasound
Exercise	Relaxation training	Other (Specify)
Herbal medicine	Surgery	

C. Please list ALL MEDICATIONS you CURRENTLYtake, including nonprescription
medications and herbal formulas:

Name of drug   Dose   Frequency

Please list PAIN MEDICATIONS you have taken in the PAST:

Name of drug   Dose   Frequency   Effectiveness

Are you allergic to any medication (including local anesthetic), latex, or shellfish?

Drug   Type of reaction

Please check any past or present medical conditions that apply to you:

___ Angina   ___ Kidney disease   ___ Seizures   ___ Arthritis
___ Heart attack   ___ Hepatitis   ___ Stroke   ___ Depression
___ Heart failure   ___ Ulcers   ___ Cancer   ___ Other:
___ Palpitations   ___ Esophagitis   ___ Back pain
___ Pacemaker   ___ Diabetes   ___ Bleeding problems
___ Lung disease   ___ Hypertension   ___ Thyroid disease

List ALL previous surgeries with dates:

D. What is your height? _____ Current weight? _____

Do you smoke? _____ If yes, how many packs/years? _____

Do you drink alcohol? _____ If yes, how much? _____

Do you use recreational drugs? _____

Are you currently employed? _____ Occupation: _____

If unemployed, for how long? _____ Is this due to a pain condition? _____

Do you receive disability benefits? _____

If so, what type? _____

Do you have a pending settlement about disability, workmen's compensation, or a legal

matter? _____Yes _____No

If yes, explain briefly:

_____

_____

_____

Please mark the area(s) of the body where your pain is on the figures below:

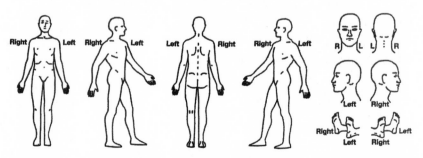

Figure 2

At Part A we gather pertinent information about the patient. This is standard stuff, except at the bottom. As you can see, I include a couple of personal questions that don't normally appear on a medical form, such as with whom in your family we are permitted to share information. Many times, a pain patient confronts personal issues she doesn't even want her other doctor to know about, let alone her family. We don't want to present any barriers to her pain cure, so we go an extra step to ensure complete privacy to maintain confidence in our program.

I also ask, "With whom do you live?" I don't really care whether you live with a lover, a college roommate, or a married man. If I find a patient is happily married with two children, however, and I see her mother also lives in the house, this tells me a little more about her potential stress level. If I see a car-accident victim who lives with no one, this tells me something about his support structure at home. No other medical specialty must address stress and emotional support as much as pain management. In my practice, it is vital.

Finally, the Painbuster Profile inquires about a personal faith system that helps you cope with pain. Anywhere else, I suppose, this type of question would be considered unconstitutional. In my practice, I resolve the pain syndromes of all patients, whether the patient is a "believer" or not. I suppose you could say that I ask this question because I like to know all the other healing "practitioners" involved in this patient's care, including God, Allah, the Buddha, or whoever. I have found that, in many cases, faith can help relieve the stress of a pain patient. More than that, I want to design a program that makes the patient most comfortable. The Painbuster program does not require any divine intervention, but having this information reveals a little more about "with whom" this patient resides.

At Part B of the profile, I want to know about the origin and life span of the pain. As we have already reviewed, some pains change into other types of pain, especially if the pain lingers more than a couple of weeks. What began as a bruised muscle from a bike injury might develop into a shooting pain down your arm, for example. If you've had pain for several weeks, then we are looking not only for the original cause of pain but also for the secondary pain that has most likely entered the picture. Questions about what activities make the pain worse or better also help to identify the combination of pains. Using this information, I'd compare your specific symptoms to the common ones listed under "The Six Types of Pain" (see page 26).

The pain scale tells me how we're progressing during the course of treatment. If you're at my pain center, I already know the pain is pretty bad. In fact, by the time a patient has been referred to me, his pain scale is quite high, and this from a patient who has usually recalibrated himself to a life with pain. But I use this scale as a reference point, using the patient's own estimation to gauge how much better he is feeling. On his subsequent visits, we'll refer to the scale again to measure his progress.

The information about a cane or crutches tells me how much general motion the body is capable of. It also reveals whether or not other parts of the body have had to compensate for the injury. Crutches, for example, can have the same effect on healthy muscles that an orthotic device might have. That is, even a cane can help prompt a new pain to join in the syndrome. That doesn't mean you shouldn't use one! But if you do, be sure to say so.

At Part C, a pain-management specialist gets to look behind the curtain of your pain syndrome. As I mentioned earlier, our anesthesiology training requires us to know the effects of every medication on each part of the body. We also must know how different medications interact with one another, from penicillin and cough syrup, to marijuana and Prozac. This expansive training in pharmaceuticals allows me to see if the effects of one are erasing another, or if the combination is making them both ineffective. A pain-management specialist knows which combinations are good for pain, and which ones are bad for pain. This is explained in further detail in chapter 4.

Finally, at Part D, I inquire about other lifestyle habits: smoking, drinking, job status. The questions about workmen's compensation and job disability benefits are helpful in measuring stress, in a different way than the personal data on Part A. Acknowledgment of the pain syndrome by your employer and his support in your recovery process help reduce frustration and stress. When I have this information, I can build a Painbuster program to compensate for the amount of support (or lack thereof), as is necessary for your case.

The drawings at Part D are the most important part of the questionnaire. People frequently cannot adequately describe their pain in words, but most can draw their pain with great detail and animation. This tells me where the pain is, and where it goes. A sciatica patient, for example, almost always draws a big arrow from the lower back down

to her leg. A deep ache might be drawn as a circle, carefully filled in, radiating to a whole area. Instead of giving
the physician just one piece of the puzzle to solve and letting the doctor find the other pieces, this drawing provides
all the information a doctor needs. All of the puzzle pieces
are here in the picture, and a doctor just needs to piece
them together.

You can perform much of the detective work for your
syndrome, just as I do. As you familiarize yourself with
your pain syndrome, and the rest of the Painbuster program, you will begin to feel better. The program is laid
out, step by step, over the next four chapters. When you
have empowered yourself with this information, you can
make effective decisions along with your own doctor, or
with your pain-management specialist. But you will start
to feel better immediately when you recognize the components of your pain condition, and see how we attack them
in ways that really work.

In the meantime, as you read the Painbuster program,
make yourself more comfortable. If you are in pain, these
home techniques can help you until you begin the Painbuster program.

Most injuries cause myofascial and bony pain. If you
injure yourself, the best thing to do—immediately—is to
put ice on the injury. Ice will decrease swelling, and
swelling is what causes much of the pain. Sometimes, the
swelling is worse than the injury. Ice helps return the area
to a more normal state. Put crushed ice in a plastic zipper
sandwich bag, or use anything that is in the freezer, such as
a bag of frozen vegetables. Apply this ice pack for fifteen to

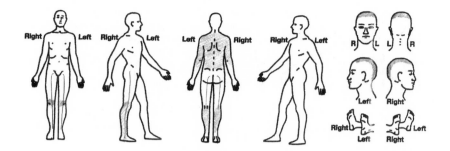

Figure 3. Fybromyalgia

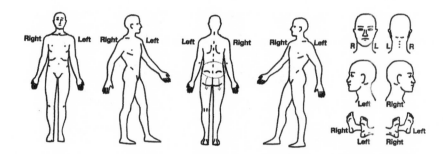

Figure 4. Lower Back Pain

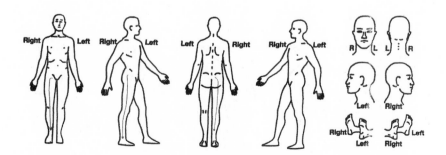

Figure 5. Herniated Disc Pain

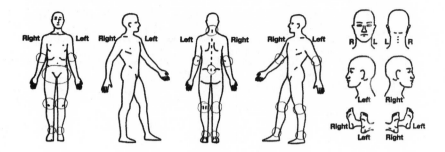

Figure 6. Arthritis

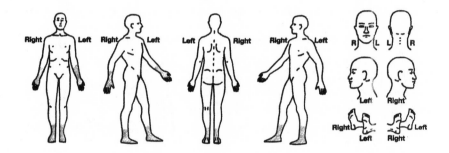

Figure 7. Diabetic Polyneuropathy

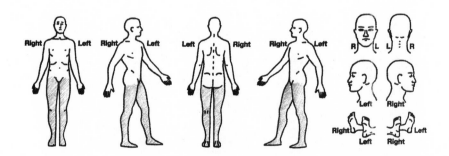

Figure 8. Vascular Pain

twenty minutes, then remove it to allow the skin some relief from the cold. Keep reapplying until swelling is reduced. Elevate the area to also help reduce the swelling. Raise the affected area so that it is above the level of your heart. Elevation helps increase drainage from the injured area toward the heart. Anti-inflammatory pain relievers, such as aspirin or Advil, are good over-the-counter remedies to take until you can seek professional treatment.

Once the ice has calmed the swelling, you might be more comfortable switching to a hot pack. If the ice was not helpful to your acute pain, heat might be the better solution for you anyway. Even a doctor admits that it is a toss-up whether heat or ice will help your particular injury—use the one that makes you most comfortable. Neither one will hurt you. When the swelling is down, it is important to move the injured part of your body. Motion will minimize any long-term damage to the area, and can indicate how serious your injury is.

Heat is helpful for general muscle aches in your neck or lower back, since it increases the blood flow to an area. It is always best to have moist heat, as opposed to the dry heat of an electric heating pad. Take a small bath towel and drizzle it with water. It should not be overly wet— about as damp as your towel after you dry off from a shower. Fold it once or twice and heat it in the microwave for at least sixty seconds. After ensuring that it is not too hot, place it over your bare skin on your aching muscles. This moist heat is much more effective than a dry heating pad.

For muscle spasms, ask someone to place a finger as a pressure point on the spot, and apply hard pressure for one minute. This person should press extremely hard, until his knuckles are white. This will break a spasm. If you're by yourself and have a spasm in your back, press your back against a doorknob or something protruding from a wall. You might even reach a specific pressure point by rolling on the floor against a tennis ball. Press against this spasm very hard, for one minute.

The next step in the Painbuster program reveals the secrets of traditional and nontraditional medication combinations and how they work—and don't work—on each type of pain.

CHAPTER 3

Pain Soup:
Oral Medications

Step Two: Combat the Pain from Every Angle

There is not yet one simple pill that can cure chronic pain. However, there are particular combinations of medication that come very close. This chapter will review what the different types of medications are and how they work together to attack pain effectively.

The body was designed to heal itself. Most pain will go away on its own, given enough time. My goal, however, is to hasten the process, or "temporize" it. No one wants to spend an extra moment in pain, if it can be avoided. There are other benefits to making the healing process go more quickly. Once pain settles in, the body immediately begins to lose strength and flexibility; physical movement can become extremely difficult. It is much easier to halt pain and, just as important—the side effects of pain—when you can stop them before they get very far.

Even a herniated disc—something quite common, and becoming even more so among gym-going baby boomers—will heal itself without treatment. But that healing process takes about five years. Herniated (from the Latin for "rupture") discs, also known as "slipped" discs, occur when the gelatinous discs between vertebrae pop out of their exterior membranes, like well-roasted marshmallows. Most herniated discs don't cause any pain at all. In fact, many people right now are walking around with no idea that they have one. But when a herniated disc sticks out into a nerve, you most certainly feel pain. A *lot* of pain. That means you have two choices: You can wait for the disc to heal and endure years of unnecessary agony, or you can eradicate the pain and restore mobility while the disc heals itself quickly, without the inevitable stress caused by the pain itself. To my way of thinking, the second option is really the only viable choice.

It is important to understand that temporizing the pain does not mean the cure is less complete. It's not like racing to build a house in two weeks instead of six months, where the work is shoddy and the final result will fall apart. Temporizing pain with medication and exercise in the four-step Painbuster program is safe, complete, *and* enduring. In fact, I have learned that the sooner a patient leaves the state of pain, the simpler the cure is, and the more successful. It is *better* for your body to heal quickly than to heal slowly. We don't want pain to build a nice home in your body. We want to eradicate it before the foundation is poured.

Doctors have long told patients "there's no such thing as a simple pill that can cure pain." That is still true. Aspirin, Tylenol, Advil, Aleve, and even narcotics like Percocet and morphine lose their effectiveness the longer you take them. To enhance their healing effects, I have learned how to use a combination of medications, as well as such things as acupuncture, massage, counseling, diet, and physical therapy. Pain management requires active supervision of all of the above treatments, which is why any discussion of medical options must not be made in isolation.

Once we've identified the source of the pain, we always begin treatment with the least invasive option. Acupuncture works well to eliminate pain for certain people and, most importantly, it has no side effects. As much as specialists might claim otherwise, even today, no one really knows why acupuncture works. Some say it blocks nerve impulses or sends distracting nerve impulses to the brain or increases the flow of endorphins, which are your body's natural pain relievers. We do know that needles delicately inserted into the skin attract blood flow to the area. These needles are traditionally placed along one of the twelve meridians—which are imaginary lines throughout the body. Meridians are the routes supplying the body's life flow—or "chi"—with energy. The different meridians affect different functions of the body. Since we can't *measure* this energy flow, it's not possible to definitively state that is exactly how it works. But that is how we *think* it works. And, quite often, it does.

Acupuncture is particularly effective on pain in the shoulders, neck, and head. It is superbly effective on most kinds of headaches, which can be the most difficult kind of pain to treat. Most patients need at least three, and as many as ten sessions, to feel its effects. We try three ways of inserting needles to achieve healing effects. Moxibustion is when we heat the needles before inserting them, electroacupuncture uses a small electric current through the needles, and sometimes we simply manipulate the needles and spin them to maximize their effect.

I rarely see acupuncture work as well on lower back problems, leg pain, or any pain in the lower extremities. What is also true about acupuncture, in my observation, is it either works for you, completely eradicating your pain, or it has no effect on you at all. There is not a lot of gray area with acupuncture, although I do sometimes use it in combination with other treatments for no other reason than to improve the chi. Acupuncture is a certified specialty, and you can find an acupuncturist by consulting your doctor or a local pain center.

If acupuncture is not what the patient wants, or responds to, then we move on to oral medications. This is, by far, the treatment method that works most effectively, because there are so many different options. The key to my success using oral medications with patients is that I almost never give a solitary prescription. By the time a patient comes to me, the pain condition has usually been exacerbated, taken firm root, or has already recruited other muscles and nerves to deliver pain signals to the brain. The nerve pain is now combining with a muscle spasm, perhaps. Almost every chronic pain is a combination pain and requires an assault from multiple directions. This has become a sort of personal battle cry for me, and it is worth repeating: every chronic pain is a combination pain and requires a multiple treatment plan. There is no question that by implementing a multifaceted attack, we can defeat pain every time.

I use a vast—but selective—arsenal of medications.

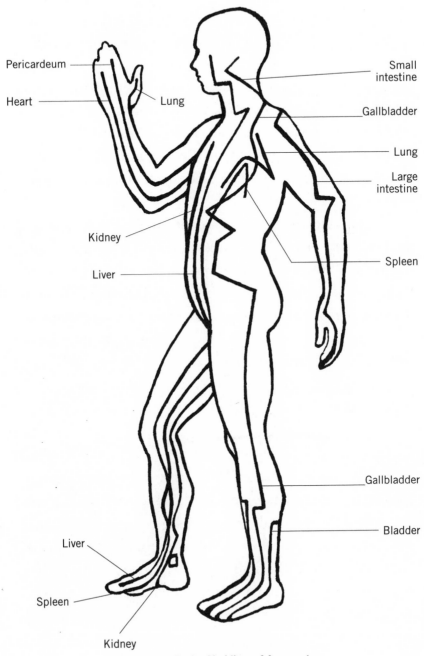

Pericardeum

Heart

Lung

Kidney

Liver

Small intestine

Gallbladder

Lung

Large intestine

Spleen

Gallbladder

Bladder

Liver

Spleen

Kidney

Figure 9: The Twelve Meridians of Acupuncture

They not only complement one another, but I have ensured that they do not conflict when they overlap. Prescribing a muscle relaxant can stop a muscle spasm, for example, but using a muscle relaxant in combination with a nonsteroidal anti-inflammatory will stop the spasm and also prevent it from expanding to adjacent areas in the body. By using such combinations, I am also able to find success with smaller doses of each medication. Although there is no simple pill that will cure pain, it is true that there are two or three, when used together, that come very close.

To provide you with the proper tools, I'll review the oral medications I have successfully used to erase pain. Every year brings many new options from the pharmaceutical labs, so I won't attempt to list all of the brand names. I think it is more important to characterize the *types* of medications now available, and explain how they work with one another to eliminate pain.

OVER-THE-COUNTER REMEDIES

Most pain patients are familiar with mild pain relievers like aspirin and acetaminophen (Tylenol), as well as one or more brands of the lower dosage nonsteroidal anti-inflammatory pain relievers called ibuprofen (Motrin IB, Advil, Aleve, and others). These work well for minor aches and pains by reducing swelling and inflammation. The differences among them are primarily their strengths and side effects.

There are several side effects for some patients who use aspirin or ibuprofen. The first involves the function of blood platelets. Platelets produce clots to stop bleeding anywhere in your body. Aspirin and ibuprofen hinder this ability in platelets, sometimes leading to excessive bruising or internal bleeding. Aspirin and ibuprofen also affect the stomach lining, as well as blood flow to major organs like the liver and kidneys. An over-the-counter remedy that works for one person may cause stomach upset in another. Acetaminophen (Tylenol) is milder than aspirin and does not have these side effects. However, Tylenol alone is not very effective against pain. It can reduce a fever well but, in general, Tylenol is best used to enhance the effect of another pain-relieving medication. Tylenol with codeine, for example, or Tylenol with oxycodone (also known as Percocet) are very safe and potent pain relievers.

I prescribe all of these nonsteroidal anti-inflammatory drugs but, because of the side effects, I do not recommend them for long-term pain syndromes such as arthritis. Fortunately, there are better over-the-counter medications for arthritis.

A new natural combination called glucosamine chondroitin sulfate complex is being used with great success to treat osteoarthritis. This is a condition where the cartilage and fluid in the joints break down, and it affects millions of people as they age. When joints become bone against bone, without any cushion, a patient experiences great pain and stiffness. I highly recommend the combination of glucosamine and chondroitin sulfates for osteoarthritis patients, because they contain the "building blocks" of cartilage.

In addition, glucosamine is an enzyme that the body needs to create cartilage. Chondroitin sulfate is derived from the shells of lobsters, crabs, and shellfish. Together, they encourage the human body to produce more cartilage and "fill in" the affected joints. Although this compound is not a pain reliever, it can bring long-lasting pain relief. I've seen it work miracles on badly affected joints: spine, knees, hips, and hands. Some arthritis patients might also get a "hyaline" injection of synthetic cartilage, which is an efficient alternative for treating an isolated joint, like an arthritic knee or elbow. This is essentially injecting the same compound directly into the joint that needs it.

Shark cartilage pills are not as effective as glucosamine and chondroitin sulfate, because the human body has to break down the shark cartilage before it can build new cartilage of its own. Glucosamine and chondroitin are already broken down, so the human body has less work to do before building new cartilage. A few years ago, you had to ask a homeopath to specially grind this compound, but now it is largely available over the counter, in health food and vitamin stores, and frequently marketed with anti-aging slogans and names like "Pain-Free." The pills take several weeks before they have a full effect and, after a couple of months of building new cartilage, a person can adjust the dose to maintain good cartilage health. If the bony pain returns, a patient can increase the glucosamine and chondroitin to a "building new cartilage dose." With forty million Americans suffering from osteoarthritis, this compound has become very popular, and deservedly so.

TOPICAL LOCAL ANESTHETICS

Some arthritis patients are helped by iontophoresis, a procedure where an electrical current helps transmit a local anesthetic through the skin to aching joints. Many topical pain relievers are effective in themselves, and they are very safe. Some creams relieve pain with an ingredient called capsaicin, which is derived from chili peppers. This is the effective ingredient of Zostrix HP cream, and it soothes nerve pain. The "heat" of Ben-Gay works in a similar manner, using methyl salicylate to increase blood flow and reduce muscle pain. For other nerve pains, we use local anesthetics called lidocaine and benzocaine, which are in products such as Solarcaine and the Lidoderm skin patch. These help relieve a variety of nerve pains, from sunburn to postherpetic neuralgia.

NONSTEROIDAL ANTI-INFLAMMATORY DRUGS (NSAIDS)

Sometimes pain management involves simple common sense. For instance, if a patient is suffering from pain caused by an inflammation, logic tells us that reducing the inflammation will stop the pain. Your body is equipped to do this itself, using hormones produced in the adrenal glands called corticosteroids. Steroids are fat-soluble organic compounds, and they reduce any inflammation in the body. Sometimes a pain syndrome needs extra steroids, however, and there are steroid drugs that are derived from both chemical and natural substances. But they are rarely prescribed in pill form to relieve pain. When a small dose is carefully injected into the precise area of inflammation, steroids are safe, quick, and effective. A small amount injected into a specific area in the body does not have the side effects of a pill, which spreads from the stomach throughout the bloodstream. In pill form, steroids can affect hormone levels, hair growth, muscle density, and menstrual cycles. Fortunately, the growing armamentarium of pain management includes an array of oral medications that are not steroids, and that are very good at reducing inflammation.

Nonsteroidal anti-inflammatory drugs like Motrin IB, Aleve, and Advil, among other brands, are ibuprofen formulas currently available in low doses as over-the-counter medications. Traditional nonsteroidal anti-inflammatory drugs, like Motrin, Naprosyn, Orudis, Feldene, Indocin, Arthrotec, and Lodine, just to name a few, are prescription drugs that require a doctor's supervision.

Nonsteroidals stop the formation of substances that cause inflammation in the body. This inflammatory agent is substance P, which is the neuromodulator (the main transmitter of pain) when you suffer a muscle injury, a crush, a workout injury, or a bony kind of pain. Sometimes, even a person in good shape who exercises a lot will get a buildup of lactic acid in the body. Lactic acid actually stimulates an accumulation of substance P, causing aching muscle pain after a workout. You get soreness from working out, you pop a Motrin. The nonsteroidal anti-inflammatory slows down substance P. The pain goes away.

Nonsteroidals have a few side effects, similar to those of aspirin, which we discussed earlier. They break down the prostaglandin throughout your body, including the lining in your stomach wall, which ordinarily protects you from getting ulcers. They also affect the platelets that control bleeding. And they can hinder blood flow to important organs like the liver and kidneys, sometimes with disastrous effect. Not long ago, a nonsteroidal anti-inflammatory called Duract was taken off the market because it was believed to have caused liver failure in a very small number of patients. Although it isn't certain that Duract caused these problems, it shows how careful the industry is about monitoring side effects. They greatly influence the kind of medical treatments we use with each patient.

For every drug that is recalled from the market, there is a new one to take its place that is even more effective. A new nonsteroidal anti-inflammatory called cyclooxygenate inhibitors, or Cox-2 inhibitors, proved so amazing that the first one was approved by the FDA after only six months of tests, in January 1999. Celecoxib was marketed by Searle under the name Celebrex, and doctors nationwide prescribed it eighty-six thousand times in the first month. Within nine months, two other variations of the Cox-2 inhibitor became available, including Merck's rofecoxib (Vioxx). These Cox-2 inhibitors produce almost none of the side effects on the kidney, liver, or stomach that traditional nonsteroidals have. And because it has fewer side effects, the Cox-2 inhibitor can be used in higher doses than the others, for longer time periods, simply providing more pain relief.

Nonsteroidal anti-inflammatories are perfect for the "weekend warrior," the man who rakes his yard, cleans his garage, and then can hardly move the next day. They work well on the rehabilitated sports injury that is still causing some discomfort. And they are frequently used by those arthritis patients who do not experience side effects. But in my Painbuster program, nonsteroidal anti-inflammatory drugs are almost never used by themselves. Most chronic pain syndromes are caused by a combination of elements, so it is rare that they will respond to nonsteroidal anti-inflammatory drugs alone. Nonsteroidal anti-inflammatories are only one part of the combination assault.

MUSCLE RELAXANTS

When muscles are stressed or injured, they often go into a protective mode—a spasm. If someone has an injured sciatic nerve or lifts too much weight, the muscles in the lower back might just lock up. Like a herniated disc, a muscle spasm will usually heal itself. But allowing it to continue spasming extends the release of substance P, which causes additional inflammation. Acupressure can stop a spasm. For extra relief, a muscle relaxant can do the trick. Sometimes the "muscle memory" extends the spasm because it trained itself to be in a spasm mode. Muscle relaxants, such as carisoprodol (Soma), baclofen (Lioresal), chlorzoxazone (Parafon Forte), and cyclobenzaprine (Flexeril) work well in relieving acute muscle injury or spasm.

As I mentioned earlier, spasms frequently spread out to other muscles, causing them to swell or spasm, too. If we used only a muscle relaxant by itself, it would unlock the original spasm but not the inflammation of the surrounding areas. For this reason, I almost always use a muscle relaxant in conjunction with a nonsteroidal anti-inflammatory, or with a medication that will stop the residual pains of a spasm. Muscle relaxants are most effective, in very small doses, when they are used in a combination.

TRICYCLIC ANTIDEPRESSANTS

I frequently borrow medications from other areas, ones that were not formulated specifically for pain relief. For instance, some tricyclic antidepressants are wonderful for nerve pain. The mediators of nerve pain are very similar to the mediators of depression. The difference is that the gateways that transmit pain are located in the spine, while the gateways transmitting depression are located in the brain. A tricyclic antidepressant drug that tweaks these mediators can decrease depression, and many of them will also tweak the mediators in the spine and alleviate pain. Antidepressants reduce nerve pain messages as effectively as a muscle relaxant stops muscle spasms.

Tricyclic antidepressants actually achieve pain management results in three ways. First, they reduce the transmission of nerve pain. Second, they clear up reactionary depression. Most pain patients have some level of depression as a reaction to pain although they may not even be aware of it. Getting rid of this depression is yet another element of the combination assault. Third, tricyclic antidepressants are sedating. Pain is frequently exacerbated when sufferers have trouble sleeping. We use this side effect to our advantage, however, by prescribing the tricyclic antidepressant to be taken just before bed-time. The patient sleeps well and feels better, too. I use antidepressants often with patients, because they are so effective and they have virtually no harmful side effects. Aside from the sedating effects, a few patients might experience dry mouth or, for older men, possible urinary retention.

Tricyclic antidepressants are used for sharpshooting nerve pains—the lightning-bolt pain of sciatica, or other large nerve pain, such as a toothache. There's a whole range of antidepressants, and they're quite distinctive. Some work fabulously for pain, better than they do for depression. Elavil, for example, is no longer used very often for depression, but it works great on pain. Other antidepressants, like Prozac, work for depression but do nothing for pain. Of course, we rarely use tricyclic antide-pressants by themselves to attack pain. Most nerve pain has another kind of pain nearby—inflammation, injury, muscle spasm. Tricyclic antidepressants are almost always used in conjunction with nonsteroidal anti-inflammatory drugs, a muscle relaxant, or even with both.

Antidepressants that are great for pain	Antidepressants that are great for depression, but not for pain
Elavil (anitryptiline)	Prozac (fluoxetine)
Pamelor (nortriptyline)	Effexor (venlafaxine)
Zoloft (sertraline)	
Paxil (paroxetine)	
Desyrel (trazodone)	

NARCOTICS

A narcotic is an opiate-based medication that treats all pain. Some of the best-known narcotics are morphine, methadone, oxycodone, and codeine. There is nothing as powerful—they simply annihilate a patient's perception of severe pain. They work because they block the transmissions of pain signals in the spinal cord—through what are known as the delta, kappa, and mu receptors—before they get to the brain. They are the fastest, strongest, and least-expensive pain relievers there are, and they work on pain in any part of the body.

No pain relievers are as efficient as narcotics. Yet no medication has a more forbidding stigma in the minds of consumers. Action movies and newspaper headlines have redefined the term *narcotics* for many people. Rather than associating narcotics with safe, effective relief for pain, people envision kilos of heroin or cocaine, street addicts, contraband trafficking, and police vice squads. This is unfortunate, because if people knew how well narcotics relieved physical agony, they would help us provide a more positive message to those who really need them. When used properly, narcotics are a safe and potent weapon against pain.

I once had a patient who was a grandmother in her eighties, Elizabeth G., whose arthritis was so bad she could hardly walk. We tried a variety of treatments, and the one that really worked for her was methadone. We put her on five milligrams, twice a day—a very small dose. Within a week, her pain was almost gone, and without a single side effect. Elizabeth felt better than she had in a very long time. She even felt good enough to go to her bridge club, which she hadn't done in two years. Her friends flocked around her and asked her what she had done to recover so much mobility and good health. When Elizabeth uttered the word *methadone*, her friends recoiled and scolded her for being foolish. They responded as if she were a drug addict. Elizabeth felt so humiliated, she stopped taking the medication that had helped her so much. Her pain returned. She stopped going to the bridge club. I felt terrible for her. But I know she feels even worse.

Sometimes even doctors inadvertently stigmatize the use of narcotics. State and federal drug enforcement agencies routinely monitor doctors' prescriptions of narcotics, so some doctors—perhaps subconsciously—prescribe doses that are simply too low. Doctors have been known to lose their medical licenses for giving proper doses to patients disabled by chronic pain. One government agency unfamiliar with a case might deem the patient's dose too high, much to the dismay of the doctor, who loses his license, and of the patient, who loses the only means of controlling her pain.

In truth, narcotics are safe, and they level the playing field. They do so by mimicking endorphins, enkephalins, and dynorphins, which are the body's own natural painkillers. Endorphins make all activity relatively painless: climbing stairs, riding a horse, even running twenty-six miles in a marathon without feeling incredible agony. When used appropriately, in low doses, narcotics allow your body to feel the effects of "extra endorphins." They eliminate the chronic pain, but not other, normal pains. If a patient taking narcotics cuts his head or burns his finger, for example, he will feel it as much as anyone else does.

The narcotic is so consumed by the act of pain relief, there is nothing extra left, not even a little "high."

There are two kinds of narcotics—short-acting ones and long-acting ones. It is important to distinguish between them to treat a patient's individual ailment correctly. Percocet (oxycodone with Tylenol) is one brand of short-acting narcotic. It is probably the most common narcotic prescription, and it's perfect for minor surgery pain, intermittent pain, or an acute injury pain that is not chronic.

For pain that is present twenty-four hours a day, it is always preferable to use a long-acting narcotic, such as OxyContin. Like Percocet, OxyContin is also a compound of oxycodone, but in a sustained-release format. Long-acting narcotics are not stronger, they are just released much more slowly into the body, allowing for a more steady delivery of the pain reliever. Here are some brands of long-acting narcotics my patients use successfully to eliminate chronic pain:

Brand name	Generic name
OxyContin	oxycodone
Kadian	morphine
Oramorph	morphine
MS Contin	morphine
Dolophine	methadone, which is not really a sustained-release medication, but a bioactive one that breaks down in the body and has an organic time-release effect all its own

Brand name	Generic name
Duragesic	a transdermal "patch" containing fentanyl
Actiq	a "lollipop" for adults that contains fentanyl, for trauma pain that breaks through normal narcotics

In a recent study of twenty-five thousand pain patients who were using one of these narcotics, only seven of them had become addicted to them. Narcotics are a miracle pain reliever, but they do have side effects. The drawbacks to narcotics might be confusion, constipation, dependence, and withdrawal when stopping the drug. These are serious side effects but, with proper pain management, all of them can be avoided. Tapering the dosage over several weeks, for instance, will enable your body to return to its normal production of endorphins, preventing the ill effects of withdrawal. If a patient finds that the narcotic makes him sleepy, we sometimes add a slight stimulant such as Ritalin to the combination. This raises alertness and has no more ill effects on the body than the addition of a buffered coating does on aspirin. If a patient suffers from constipation instead, we might overlap a stool softener such as Senokot. All of these combinations are very safe. A doctor monitors every pain patient on narcotics therapy, so he or she will not encounter the side effects of narcotics.

Certain patients may not be able to take narcotics, because the side effects are too overpowering, yet they still need something more than a nonsteroidal anti-inflammatory to control pain. We have another alternative, which is a synthetic opioid called Ultram (tramadol). Ultram has pain-relieving effects similar to those of narcotics combined with a tricyclic antidepressant. It affects the central nervous system as well as brain chemistry to relieve pain.

One of the state-of-the-art breakthroughs in narcotics treatment focuses on new methods of delivering the narcotics. Instead of being ingested through pills, narcotics can be targeted directly to the spinal cord, where all of the narcotic receptors are located. This means a far lower dosage can bring powerful pain relief, with almost none of the side effects. One delivery method that safely administers narcotics to pain patients is the intrathecal infusion device. Intrathecal means "inside the dura," which is the sac that holds all the spinal nerves. The intrathecal infusion device is a pump, the size of a hockey puck. It is implanted unobtrusively in the abdominal wall and linked, via internal catheter, to the exact spot where the pain receptors are. With one-thousandth of the normal dose, the narcotic is delivered more efficiently, right where it needs to be. One milligram of morphine, administered intrathecally, is as effective as one thousand milligrams taken orally. Every few weeks the pump can be refilled in a doctor's office, and the patient can continue a normal, functional life without pain, and without any of the side effects of oral medication.

Jamie D. was a seventeen-year-old terminal cancer patient with an aggressively growing tumor in her spine. In addition to her physical problems, Jamie also had some troubled relationships with people she loved, and she wanted to come to terms with them before she died. Jamie wanted some quality time, for herself and for her family and friends. My goal with this patient was simply to get her pain under control, using the most effective and comfortable method. I provided Jamie with an intrathecal infusion device, which slowly pumped the narcotic directly to the nerves in the spinal cord. This eliminated her incapacitating pain and maintained her clarity of mind, so Jamie was able to comfortably resolve important issues at the end of her life.

When other medications fail, this one almost always works. Most of my narcotics patients are not terminal patients. They are active, healthy people who have regained their normal lives. When used properly, narcotics can work forever without affecting the mind, and without any side effects at all. Like all medications, we use narcotics in low doses and in combination with other drugs such as NSAIDs. They are our best weapon against chronic pain.

ORAL ANTIARRHYTHMICS

Antiarrhythmics are usually prescribed for heart patients who have arrhythmia, which is an abnormal heartbeat. These medications prevent aberrations of the electrical transmission through the heart, which could stop the heart from beating. Antiarrhythmics like Mexitil (mexiletine, an oral form of the local anesthetic called lidocaine) can also be used to treat small nerve pain. Mexitil is very effective on burning-type sensations or numbness, like the burning pain caused by frostbite. Some diabetics who have the stocking-glove distribution of pain through their hands and feet are helped tremendously by antiarrhythmics. Many of our patients are surprised to learn this because, until very recently, antiarrhythmics have not normally been prescribed as a medication for diabetes.

Mark J. was a forty-seven-year-old man who was newly diagnosed with diabetes. He had the classic stocking-glove, burning pain in his hands, feet, and lower legs. Mark's diabetes was being successfully treated by his endocrinologist, but the pain was still making it difficult for him to function normally. They had tried everything, including narcotics, to no avail. His endocrinologist sent Mark to me, to see if I could help him. After I examined him, I prescribed Mexitil. Within a few days, Mark's pain was greatly diminished. We then started him on an exercise routine and helped him with a new sugar-free, low-fat diet. At last he was able to walk around and use his hands comfortably. You could almost say that Mark is in better shape now than he was before he developed diabetes. Of course, he is continuing his diabetic treatments with his endocrinologist, who had been unaware of the effects of Mexitil to relieve diabetic pain. Now, Mark is pain-free, and without the despair associated with pain, which might have further exacerbated his condition.

ANTISEIZURE MEDICATIONS

Neuropathic pain, or nerve pain, simply doesn't have any specific medication of its own. It is the most difficult pain to treat with any medications other than injections or narcotics. Most of the agents we use to control nerve pain are borrowed from elsewhere, like tricyclic antidepressants. We've learned that anticonvulsants (antiseizure medications) also work well to eliminate nerve pain.

Epileptics take drugs like Neurontin (gabapentin) or Tegretol (carbamazepine) to prevent seizures. These medications reduce the firing of nerves in general. In low doses, Neurontin and Tegretol are also wonderful for burning, aching, or sharp pains that are localized in one area. These medications know how to chemically locate and shut down the firing of small nerve pains, wherever they are in the body. Patients who have chronic nerve pain, like trigeminal neuralgia, benefit greatly from anticonvulsants. They work better on small nerve pains than on large nerve pain like sciatica.

Pain Soup

Combining these medications is almost always quite safe, if done under a doctor's supervision, and I have found combining is essential to achieving a complete pain cure. I cannot stress enough that pain is always a combination of ailments and is best attacked with a combination of forces. Treating chronic pain is not as simple as treating an infection, where a doctor might say, "You have this bacteria, which causes these symptoms, and which are cured by this antibiotic." Pain is much more an individual problem, and it presents itself as a puzzle to solve. Solutions that work for one person may not work for another. It's my job to help each person solve that puzzle and restore his quality of life. I call the family of combinations Pain Soup. The recipe is not the same for each patient, but it can always cure what ails her.

Cheryl P. was an athletic, forty-something business owner in New York City. She had an active lifestyle and worked out at a gym several times a week. Three years ago, while weight lifting at her gym, she felt something "click" in her back. She'd been through a similar injury before. Cheryl was confident she could ride out the pain and get herself back into shape.

Weeks passed, and Cheryl's pain got worse. She couldn't stand without agony for more than five minutes, and sitting was no better. She took large doses of Advil and stopped going to the movies or even out to lunch. Cheryl spent two years seeking professional treatment for her pain, from a variety of doctors. She also tried massage therapy, yoga, chiropractors, Pilates, kinesiology, and hypnosis. Nothing helped. While consulting yet another orthopedist, Cheryl was finally referred to my office.

I diagnosed myofascial pain with an acute exacerbation. In other words, Cheryl's original lumbar disc injury had been made worse by muscle spasm which, in turn, had also recruited other muscles to hurt. Along the way, these aching muscles trained all the nearby nerves to repeatedly send pain messages to her brain. I prescribed the tricyclic antidepressant Elavil for Cheryl, so her pain mediators would slow down. After all, they had been sending pain messages to her brain for two long years. The antidepressant effects of Elavil stopped the pain messages from getting delivered to the brain. I also prescribed Motrin for Cheryl, to break down the substance P that had inflamed the muscles around the original injury. Although those two drugs helped Cheryl immensely, she was still not completely pain-free a couple of weeks later. So we added a muscle relaxant to her treatment. After taking Lioresal with the Elavil and the Motrin, each of them in a very small dose, Cheryl's pain disappeared.

As soon as Cheryl could comfortably move her body, she began a personalized exercise program to strengthen her muscles. Rehabilitation allowed us to decrease the medications as she got better. After several months of treatment and physical therapy, Cheryl's chronic pain disappeared almost completely, and she recovered her normal, active life.

All of these medications are more effective at stopping pain when they are used in a combination like this, where the muscle relaxant controls the afflicted muscle, while the nonsteroidal stops the pain of inflammation, and the antidepressant calms the nerves. With a combination like that, we should be able to achieve at least a 75 percent reduction in pain, if not 100 percent in every patient. When the pain is under control, then we start specific movement therapy to strengthen the muscles and to reeducate the body to move in a more normal way. This is the only way to prevent the pain from coming back. The medication eliminates pain, but does not prevent it from returning—only physical therapy does that. Medications enable the patient to begin the physical therapy without pain.

One of the many advantages of pain centers is that, for patients who have literally tried everything else with their family doctor, my focused specialty allows me to maximize the effects of traditional medications in an ever-changing variety. I can also determine the very best new drugs that come onto the market every day. You have an entire armamentarium with all the different ways to treat pain. There are constant innovations in pain research, so every day your list of options grows longer: someone discovers a new application for an established drug, or creates a new medication that eliminates pain more effectively than others. Neurex is developing a drug that uses the venom of the conus sea snail to mute pain pathways in the brain. Abbott Laboratories will soon seek approval for ABT-594, a pain reliever derived from the poison of an Ecuadorean frog that is seventy times more potent than morphine.

We can all look forward to these innovations, but the simple truth is we already possess the necessary medications to cure pain. Your doctor can help you determine which of these medications, if any, might help your chronic pain. Some of the medication combinations may seem unusual, but when your doctor observes their effects, he or she should be more than comfortable overlapping these prescriptions. Your doctor may even know about a new medication with pain-relieving characteristics that I have not yet found. By thinking creatively about the effects of certain medications (and weighing their side effects, of course), and by thinking like a pain-management specialist, and by paying attention to the clues and eliminating the contradictions, you and your doctor may even design a whole new combination that eliminates your pain. There was a time when Rogaine (minoxidil) was strictly a little-known hypertension medication. Now, Rogaine is a hugely popular topical treatment for hair growth. Aspirin once was used only for fevers—now it's taken to prevent heart attacks.

One day soon, I hope, a similar transition in the consumer's mind may take place with antidepressants, narcotics, or antiseizure medications for pain management. For the moment, my colleagues and I continue to call these unique pain-relief combinations "pain soup." The list of ingredients might change, but I can always find one that makes a patient safe, comfortable, and one step closer to physical therapy. I can even deliver medications in a way that brings immediate relief before the patient leaves my office.

CHAPTER 4

More Pain Soup: Injection Therapy

Judith Z., a thirty-two-year-old executive in Manhattan, was in a taxicab on her way to an important presentation. She was confident and well prepared, knowing that this would be an important day for the future of her career. Her thoughts were interrupted when another car rear-ended her cab at a stoplight. Although no one was seriously injured, a muscle spasm took hold in Judith's neck. As she looked around for another cab, the spasm grew worse. Judith thought about her presentation, which was to begin in ninety minutes. The spasm grabbed her even harder by the neck.

Within twenty minutes, Judith found her way to my office and requested emergency treatment. She couldn't turn her neck at all, but moved her whole torso instead. I asked her when she was slated to give her presentation, and I noticed her shoulders contracted further every time the word *presentation* was mentioned. At this point, stress was doing the most damage to her neck. Fortunately, we were able to help Judith. A trigger-point injection of a tiny amount of steroid combined with a local anesthetic calmed the muscle immediately. She was able to relax and move normally within fifteen minutes. We gave her prescription Motrin to prolong the pain relief and sent her off in good spirits to deliver her big presentation.

You don't have to be an emergency case to receive immediate pain relief. We frequently jump-start pain treatment with an injection of pain medication right into the affected area. This brings virtually instant relief.

With oral medications, the pain reliever is absorbed into the stomach, picked up by the bloodstream, and disseminated throughout the whole body. With an injection, the medication is delivered locally, right where the pain is, without flowing to parts of the body that don't need it. An injection prevents the drug from being diluted as it travels to the injured spot. Therefore, an injection is simply more potent. This means we can use a significantly smaller dose of medication when we're using it in an injection. Not all pain problems are focused enough to be cured by a targeted injection. But one of the basic tenets of pain management is to deliver medication in the smallest amount necessary, to the most specific area possible.

Sometimes, patients are hesitant about injection therapy. I like to use the analogy of another irritating scenario. Imagine an annoying black fly, buzzing endlessly around your house. You can solve the problem with a simple flyswatter, or you can solve the problem by bombing the whole house with pesticide. The preferred choice, in this instance, is the flyswatter. Of course, some patients would claim that they have a third choice: to leave the annoying fly alone, pretending it doesn't bother them, until their composure is slowly shredded to pieces. If your pain is centered around a single area, then the most efficient treatment is in the precision of an injection.

Injection therapy is almost always used in conjunction with oral medications. Injections give the medications a head start, which is usually much appreciated by the patient. For example, a patient with a muscle spasm in his lower back would normally receive oral medications to reduce the spasms and inflammation. But sometimes his spasm might be in a place that will benefit from a quick injection that hastens the effects of all the medications.

There are many different syndromes, such as a muscle spasm, that respond well to injection therapy. The most common places for painful muscle spasms are along the vertebrae, from the neck to the lower back. For a spasm, I might recommend one of the most common types of injection, the trigger-point injection. This refers to the injection going into the precise area that is triggering the pain. If I can feel a muscle spasm with my hand, I know this spasm can be successfully stopped with a trigger-point injection.

Trigger-Point Injections

The simplest type of this injection is called "dry needling." It is just what it sounds like—an empty needle is placed through the skin into the spasmodic muscle. The needle is manipulated into the muscle several times. The irritation of the needle going in and out of a muscle will often stop the spasm. This is a similar concept to the one used by practitioners of acupressure and acupuncture.

The next least invasive approach to the muscle spasm is injecting a harmless fluid into the area to stop the spasm. This could be one of several innocuous fluids, such as normal saline or salt water, injected into the painful area. Like dry needling, the needle stimulus irritates the muscle, and the expansion of fluid into the muscle helps to break the spasm. Saline is considered less invasive than injections of medications because there is a very small likelihood of allergic reaction. However, without additional medications inside a trigger-point injection, the chances of sustained relief are not great. Dry needling or saline injection can reverse a muscle spasm, but it can't always prevent it from returning.

The next more aggressive injection therapy contains a local anesthetic, such as lidocaine (Xylocaine). The local anesthetic has a multitude of effects on a muscle. First, it numbs the whole area by decreasing the transmission of pain impulses through the surrounding nerves. Second, it numbs the pain generator itself—the muscle spasm—and erases the pain. Finally, the local anesthetic has a volume effect, like the saline, simply enlarging the muscle until it is forced to relax.

The effect of a local anesthetic in a trigger-point injection depends largely on the type of drug used and the location of the injury. The longest-lasting available anesthetic, such as bupivicaine, lasts four to six hours. And even with a trigger-point injection, some of the medication is immediately picked up by the bloodstream and carried elsewhere, to the liver, for example, where it is broken down and eventually eliminated from the body. In most cases, the local anesthetic can relax the muscle long enough for it to return to its normal state. But if the muscle does not relax long enough to reset itself in a healthy state, the spasm will be back when the local anesthetic wears off. This might happen four to six hours later, when the patient is at home and there is no one there to treat the returning spasm. Therefore, we complement a trigger-point injection with oral medications that help keep the spasm away. This might be an oral muscle relaxant and a nonsteroidal anti-inflammatory medication, a combination that extends the effects of the injection. In fact, when we take the time to start oral medications a couple days before the injection, they provide a background of muscle relaxation that makes a trigger-point injection even more lasting and effective.

Local anesthetics such as lidocaine are the most common substances injected into a muscle spasm. As with most drugs, there is a slight possibility of allergic reaction, and a limit to how much local anesthetic can be used at any one time. This is based on the patient's weight. If the dose is too high, there is a high risk of toxicity, which could lead to a seizure or even paralyze the heart. The toxicity is not cumulative, in other words, most of the anesthetic will break down and leave the body within twelve hours of an injection. Placing the needle in the correct place is imperative. If an injection misses the muscle and enters the bloodstream, for example, it not only increases the chances of an adverse reaction, but the medication is carried away without any effect on the muscle spasm.

Another medication that is commonly added to a local anesthetic injection is a steroid compound. The steroids we use are in a completely different class than the ones used by athletes to build muscle. A pain specialist's steroid compound, such as the one called Kenalog, is the most potent anti-inflammatory drug there is. A steroid has, essentially, two effects on the human body. One is called glucocorticoid action, which changes the body's hormones and their normal interactions with glucose. The second effect of steroids is the mineralocorticoid action, which is the balancing of minerals (primarily salts) in the body, and the reduction of inflammation. Reducing inflammation is the primary goal when using a steroid compound in an injection. Even in a muscle spasm, the very act of spasming causes muscles to swell even more. In addition, inflammation damages surrounding tissues, causing them to swell also. Anti-inflammatories will return a muscle to its normal relaxed state.

Jerry B. lifted a heavy carton of books and injured his lower back. A small portion of his muscle was pulled, and probably slightly torn. We call this an avulsing injury. The avulsion caused immediate spasming in Jerry's other back muscles. In addition, the extra work of spasming caused even more swelling. A small amount of steroid injected into this area reduced all the swelling and hastened Jerry's healing process.

Steroids are almost always used in conjunction with a local anesthetic. The local anesthetic treats the spasm and forces it to stop spasming. The steroid reduces swelling, enhances the effects of the anesthetic, and hastens the healing process once the spasm has stopped.

There are a large number of steroid preparations available for trigger-point injections, and they have almost no side effects. The risks are small, but it is important to work with a physician who has experience with trigger-point injections. If the steroid is injected by accident into the skin or fat, it will cause those tissues to die, permanently changing the skin pigment or surface. Doctors know to use only a small amount, injected right where it needs to be. Athletes who use anabolic steroids for muscle enhancement or patients who use steroids to reduce asthma or lupus use far greater doses than a pain patient does, in addition to using a different class of drugs. There is nothing to fear from the steroids injected by an experienced doctor to alleviate pain.

The trigger-point injection is hardly invasive at all. The needle is the smallest type that still allows fluid to pass through it. The doctor identifies the target with his hand, cleans the area with an antiseptic solution, and places the needle through the skin to the target. This involves a tiny pain that quickly disappears. Anticipation of the injection is usually worse than the procedure itself. Recovery takes about fifteen minutes, by which time the pain at the trigger-point will be gone, or much reduced, leaving behind a temporary dull ache.

Epidural Space Injections

Another common type of injection therapy is the epidural steroid injection, which is also called an epidural block. The epidural space is inside the spinal column, but just outside ("epi") the sac that holds the spinal cord (the "dura"). The epidural space extends from the base of the skull to the tailbone, and it is filled with fat. All of the body's nerves pass through this space as they spread from the spinal cord out into the body. These spinal nerves instruct the muscles what to do with their strength, and they also give input to the brain about what they sense is happening in the body. These nerves in the spinal column can become inflamed or irritated by a number of causes. One of the most common irritations to the spinal nerves is a herniated disc. This is when a gelatinous disc between vertebrae has popped out, pressing on the sac that holds the spinal column.

The location of the epidural steroid injection depends on where the pain is. If the nerve pain is in an upper extremity, such as the wrist or arm, then the steroid injection would go into the neck area of the epidural space. For pain in the lower back or legs, the injection would go into the epidural space of the lower spine. An injection into the epidural space allows pain-relieving medication to get as close as possible to these irritated nerves, without injecting them into the nerves themselves, which might damage them.

The variety of medications available for epidural injections increases every day. The epidural injection usually contains a steroid solution, with or without a local anesthetic. The steroid has an anti-inflammatory effect on the nerves, reducing the swelling and thus reducing the pain. One common steroid compound, Kenalog, works well in all epidural injections. Narcotics work well in the epidural space, because the natural opiate receptors in the body are in this space also, and they react to even tiny doses of injected narcotics. Sometimes, as with oral medications,

we borrow injection medications from other fields of medicine. For example, clonidine is an oral medication that
prevents hypertension. As an injection, clonidine is very
effective in the epidural space, with analgesic qualities
that safely reduce pain. If we know the drug is safe,
approved by the Federal Drug Administration, and without adverse side effects, there's no reason a qualified pain-
management specialist can't use this drug if it relieves
chronic pain.

For an epidural injection, the physician determines the
"landmarks" with her hands. When the entry point is identified, the area is sometimes numbed with a small injection
of local anesthesia. Injections into the epidural space can be
done by feeling the change of resistance in the needle tip, or
by using X-ray guidance, whichever the doctor prefers. Once
the correct space is identified, the medication is injected and
the needle is removed. After a short recovery, the entire procedure should take no more than twenty minutes. The
epidural steroid injection will provide increasing pain relief
over the course of two or three days. After about five days, if
the pain relief is not complete, the patient and doctor may
decide to repeat the procedure. It is rare that even the worst
pains require more than three epidural blocks.

The physician who administers injections does not
need a special license to use epidural needles, but you
should find a doctor who is experienced in such injections,
either in an office or in a hospital. There are two possible
complications from epidural injections, which your doctor
should know. One is placing the injection into the wrong
area, and the other is risk of infection, both of which can
be avoided when every effort is made to prevent them.

Also, if the needle goes too far in the wrong place, the tiny hole may not close immediately after the needle is removed, causing fluid to leak from this hole. This leaking fluid is the same fluid that keeps the brain afloat. With the loss of this support, the brain is pulling on other supports. This patient might suffer what is known as a spinal headache, or postdural puncture headache, which can last for several days. This spinal headache is ever present when the patient is standing up, but goes away when the patient lies down. It is important to have an epidural steroid injection done by experienced hands, because such doctors know the spinal cord area better than any other doctor.

Nerve Block Injections

There is one more type of injection therapy. It is the one we call the "nerve block" or "advanced block." This is not to be confused with injections that use alcohol or botulism toxin (Botox). A Botox injection is an advanced procedure and does not fall into the normal realm of injection therapy. Advanced procedures are described in chapter 8. The nerve block is similar to an epidural injection, but it is applied in the specific nerve centers, rather than in the epidural space. Sometimes the nerve block injection will go into a generalized area of nerves, where the exact source of pain is not obvious. The nerve block might also go into a sympathetic nerve.

The sympathetic nervous system is comprised of several different junctions of nerves throughout the body, such as the lower back and the abdomen. Each of these nerve groups is called a plexus, and each serves a different part of the body. Nerve ailments such as causalgia and complex regional pain syndrome (which used to be known as reflex sympathetic dystrophy) are often diagnosed by using temporary nerve blocks. If the pain is not relieved, then these diagnoses can be eliminated.

Nerve blocks are usually performed with X-ray guidance, and with some level of sedation, so they are rarely uncomfortable for the patient. A temporary nerve block of local anesthetic lasts for a couple of hours, after which the doctor and patient will evaluate the extent of its pain relief. Careful records must be kept in order to weigh the benefits of this procedure, as it is usually one of the last steps before more invasive treatments, advanced procedures, or surgery.

Steroids reduce inflammation, returning the tissue to its original condition. If inflammation is causing the pain, then a steroid injection will eliminate the cause of this pain. A nerve block injection of local anesthetic will relieve pain only as long as the drug's effects last—a few hours. Local anesthetics and steroids are usually used together in this injection because, as with all injections, a smaller dose of each makes them safe and more effective.

Injection therapy is one of the safest ways to treat many types of pain. Even so, some patients prefer not to have an injection. This is fine, as long as there are oral medications that will bring about the same results. Oral medications simply take a couple of weeks longer than injections to reach the same level of pain relief. The goal of both the injections and oral medications is to eliminate the pain so we can reach the next step in the program. When you are pain-free, you can move properly. That's when we go for the permanent pain cure in Step Three: physical therapy.

CHAPTER 5

Moving Away from Pain

Step Three: Physical Therapy Is the Cure

Years, months, or even a few days of pain take a heavy toll on the body. Pain affects not just the injured area, but the healthy parts, too. Immediately after the original injury, the body recalibrates itself into a revised state of functionality, using a slightly different posture or weight shift. This change is quickly embedded in the muscle memory as normal. The healthy parts pick up on the change, compensating for the pain until they start to hurt, too. The body adjusts once again, this time causing further unnatural motion and pain. For example, Aaron, a thirty-five-year-old man, twisted his left knee in a bad golf swing. To compensate for the pain, he started limping, putting extra weight and stress on his right knee. His whole body was now moving with a completely different dynamic. After only a day or two, the right knee began to protest the abnormal stress—it began to hurt, and was still operating abnormally to compensate for the pain in the left knee. Now, both knees hurt. So Aaron's body compensated again, only this time in the hips and pelvis, to lessen the stress on both knees. After only a few days, this kind of domino effect can erase your body's memory of all normal, pain-free motion.

Only one thing can stop this degenerative process and block chronic pain: physical therapy. This is any supervised exercise program that returns the body to its normal condition, whatever it was like before the pain began. Physical therapy (PT) frequently returns the body to even better condition than before the injury. If injections or medications are used without physical therapy, the patient will have the pain reversed. But PT maintains the long-term success that the drugs helped achieve. Medications block the pain, but physical therapy heals the body.

When the medicated patient enters a relatively pain-free state, she begins a series of customized exercises she couldn't do before, when she was in pain. These exercises, determined by her type of injury or pain, rebuild body strength and stabilize the injured area. Equally important, physical therapy reteaches the entire body how to move in the normal ways it was designed to do. It eliminates the compensation that was embedded in the muscle memory. Returning the body to normal motion gives the pain nowhere to go, except out of the body completely.

It is crucial that you complete Steps One and Two before beginning physical therapy. Doing any exercise while still in pain is counterproductive—it will actually do more harm than good. Some physicians have made the mistake of sending patients out for physical therapy after an injury, without first providing enough pain relief. If you are still in pain, physical therapy will not help. If it hurts to do an exercise, you'll do it incorrectly. It's normal in physical therapy to feel a few aches after exercise, since you're working old muscles that are out of shape and producing lactic acid. But if you're hurting while you're in motion, then your motion is going to change. Within a couple of days, you might only do the exercises that don't hurt and skip the ones that cause pain, even though those are usually the most important exercises. Then what happens is that any excuse not to go to PT becomes a good excuse. You do less and less, until all you're doing is stretching and getting massages. Rehabilitation has essentially stopped, but the problem is still there. Without progress, you'll see little point in continuing the physical therapy. Plus, it hurts, so any excuse will stop you from doing it. It's nobody's fault, but this rehab has now come to a crashing halt. This is why it's important to use medication therapy *before* beginning physical therapy.

Marcy O. was a fibromyalgia patient in her thirties whose pain was well controlled by oral medications. She attended physical therapy during the first couple of weeks she was out of pain, mostly to humor her doctor (me). Marcy felt so good during this period, she determined she was cured of her chronic pain syndrome and didn't really need physical therapy. After a couple of weeks, she had not yet returned to the stage of normal flexibility and function, but she stopped coming in for therapy for nearly two months. When I saw her again, she had developed shin splints from her swing dancing lessons, and then sprained her ankle in a skiing accident. These new pains depressed her, and she came to me for new medications. Marcy didn't need new medications; what she needed was the physical therapy she had skipped. The joy of being pain-free had seduced her into physical activity for which she wasn't ready.

Physical therapy in pain management is much different than physical therapy after an accident, surgery, or stroke. Those ailments have less to do with pain than with returning normal body functions. In fact, standard physical therapy for stroke or trauma patients is rarely hampered by pain, as it is for chronic pain patients. For other patients, the structural problem has been corrected, and strengthening is the most important goal. Patient and therapist note progress with each session, and they are satisfied. Physical therapy for a pain patient is a greater challenge. The pain patient's overall condition is usually much worse than that of the postsurgical patient. Progress is slower. The body's structure has not yet been corrected— for a pain patient, this is what physical therapy will achieve. In order for a pain patient to reach recovery, the therapist must understand the distinction between this type of physical therapy and the other types for stroke or postsurgical patients. Also, the therapist must understand proper medical management for the pain patient to ensure that there is enough pain control during any movement. No physical therapy should begin until the patient has achieved a significant reduction in pain, through medication or whatever method. In today's health-care environment, there is a limit to how much physical therapy the managed-care plans will cover, so this time needs to be used wisely. Finally, patient and therapist should understand that exercises will be based on teaching the patient how to use proper techniques, so that he can continue to use them and maintain correct motions after the treatment has ended.

Physical therapy for pain management is broken down into three parts: flexibility and function, strengthening, and conditioning. These three elements must be combined—just as medications are combined—in order for the pain patient's physical therapy to be successful.

FLEXIBILITY AND FUNCTION

The first step in physical therapy is to ensure that painless movement is possible at all. Strength and condition will not return without first reaching normal flexibility and function. For example, a patient with lower back pain usually walks with a limp. You may not even notice a limp, but back pain forces this patient to use different combinations of muscles to walk. If this patient went straight to a strengthening exercise, this would fortify the limp, cementing it as part of her normal gait. This patient must first be restored with flexibility and function. She must spend time learning the correct posture for her lower back, and the appropriate way to walk.

Everyday posture and gait training are frequently overlooked by standard physical therapy, but the Painbuster program is founded on it. The lower back is like a giant joint connecting the hips and back to the knees and ankles. Proper alignment of the whole structure prevents injury to any one of them—it is the definition of the body's healthy function. And proper posture and gait stabilize the lower and upper back with flexibility and function, which is rewarded with progress throughout the rehabilitation. Then this patient can move on to strengthening exercises.

Another example of the importance of flexibility and function can be found in the shoulders and arms. The shoulder, like the hip, is a very dynamic joint. It pivots, rotates, twists, and bends. When pain restricts a shoulder joint, it can become "frozen," which restricts motion of the entire arm. Rather than simply strengthening the arm, the shoulder joint must be trained to move correctly and to regain flexibility. The arm will never return to its full range of motion unless the shoulder joint is made functional first.

When a pain syndrome starts, the first things the patient loses are flexibility and function. Therefore, once the pain is controlled, it is vital that flexibility and function be the first goals of physical therapy. This is a stage where it is most important to have supervision by a physical therapist or doctor, since this is when you are most vulnerable to injury if it is done incorrectly.

Checking Your Gait

The best way to check your gait is to get a gait analysis from a physical therapist. You can, however, make a preliminary check of your typical gait, which may allow you to determine if a professional examination and evaluation are necessary. To do so, all you'll need is a full-length mirror.

1. Walk directly toward the mirror, checking that:
   · Your knees remain straight.

- Your body displays an overall symmetry.
- Your arms swing rhythmically to counterbalance legs.
- Your hips are level.
- You feel as if you are "walking tall."

2. Walk past the mirror, checking that:
   - Your heel is the first part of your foot to make contact with the ground.
   - You "roll off" the toes, ending with the big toe.
   - Your steps are of equal length.

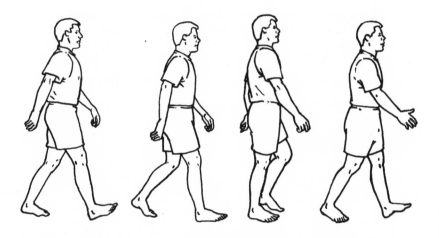

Proper Gait

Posture

In addition to walking correctly, it is important for your body to remember how to rest properly. People who have been living with a chronic pain are sometimes skewed in a slightly protective posture. Their muscles are tensed around the injured area, causing a shoulder to slump or a hip to be stressed. Even just sitting in a chair, a pain patient leans toward one side, tensing parts of her lower back.

Stand still, look in a mirror, and observe the line of your posture.

- Shoulders are back, down, and relaxed.
- Neck is straight, forming a continuous line of the spine.
- Chin is level with the ground.
- Back is straight, with pelvis slightly tucked in.
- Knees are relaxed.

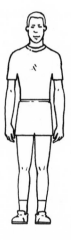

Proper standing posture
(front view)

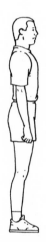

Proper standing posture
(side view)

There are several specific ways to increase flexibility and function. Begin by evaluating the affected area. Where are the weaknesses, and what is the therapy goal? Stretching increases the range of any joint or muscle. Here are some stretch routines for a pain patient, which you can start slowly. Try doing each of these ten times, every other day. Warm up beforehand, by moving slowly or even by taking a hot shower first. When they become easy for you, repeat them each ten times every day. If it hurts while you're doing any of these, stop immediately. If you feel a little sore after doing them, that's normal. Start your stretch routine slowly, but be consistent. It may not seem so, but this is the most important step to your freedom from pain.

Seated Low Back Stretch

Targets the muscles in the low back, buttocks, and shoulders.

1. Sit all the way back on a sturdy, armless chair, with your arms at your sides and your shoulders down and relaxed (the back of the chair should be straight and positioned near a wall, if possible). Keep your stomach in, small of back pressed toward the back of the chair, chin tucked, gaze forward, and head upright. Inhale.
2. Bend your trunk down, allowing your hands to reach toward the floor and your head to rest on your knees. Exhale as you stretch down. Hold the stretch for 5 to 30 seconds, breathing evenly as you

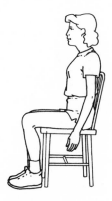
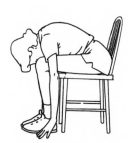

hold. Return to the starting position, uncurling slowly, one vertebra at a time, inhaling slowly as you sit up.

V-Sit Stretch

Targets the muscles in the inner thighs and low back.

1. Sit with your legs out straight and placed as far apart as possible. Keep your knees slightly bent, your stomach tight, and your neck straight to maintain good alignment. Inhale.
2. Gently lean your trunk forward between your legs. Reach forward, sliding your hands across the floor, as you attempt to touch your head to the floor. Exhale as you stretch forward. Hold the stretch for 5 to 30 seconds, breathing evenly as you hold. Return slowly to the starting position, inhaling as you sit up.

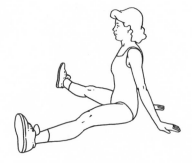 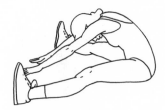

Cat Stretch

Targets the muscles in the back.

1. Kneel down on your hands and knees. Keep your chin tucked and head and neck aligned and straight. Inhale.
2. Pull your stomach and chin in as you slowly round your back up. Inhale as you round up and don't let your back sag. Hold for 5 to 30 seconds, breathing evenly as you hold. Return slowly to the starting position.

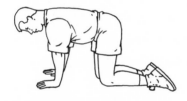 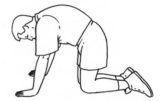

Reverse Cat Stretch

Targets the muscles in the upper and low back and abdomen.

1. Kneel down on your hands and knees. Keep your stomach in, chin tucked, and head and neck aligned and straight. Inhale.

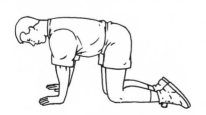 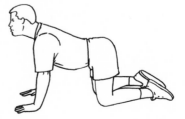

2. In the on-knees position, drop your stomach and arch your back in a reverse cat stretch position. Exhale as you stretch. Hold the stretch for 5 to 30 seconds, breathing evenly as you hold. Return slowly to the starting position.

Standing Quad Stretch

Targets the muscles in the front of the thighs and hips.

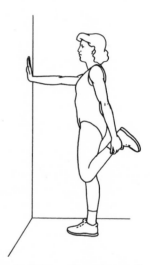

1. Stand up straight and face a wall about arm's distance away. Keep your stomach in, chin tucked, gaze forward, head upright, and knees slightly bent. Place your right palm against the wall for balance. Inhale.

2. Grasp your left ankle with your left hand and gently pull your knee backward, keeping your thighs even. (To increase the stretch, press your knee toward the floor at the same time as you press your hip slightly forward, but do not arch your back.) Exhale as you stretch. Hold the stretch for 5 to 30 seconds, breathing evenly as you hold.

3. Repeat on the opposite side.

Standing Hamstring Stretch

Targets the muscles in the back of the upper thighs, hips, and back.

1. Stand up straight, lift one leg, and place the heel of that leg on the edge of a table (or a lower surface, such as a step stool or coffee table). Bend your other knee slightly and turn your standing foot so that it's slightly pointing out (use a nearby wall or chair for support if necessary). Inhale.
2. Tighten your stomach and keep your neck straight to maintain proper alignment, then put your right hand on your right thigh and slowly lean your body forward. Exhale as you stretch. Hold the stretch for 5 to 30 seconds, breathing evenly as you hold. Return slowly to the starting position.
3. Repeat on the opposite side.

You may also do this stretch by simply putting one leg out in front, heel on the floor, and gently leaning as far forward as you can, with your back knee bent and your hands on your thighs.

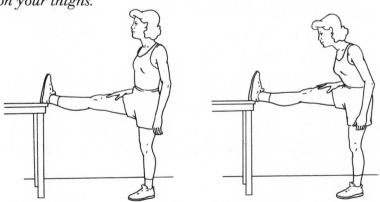

Massage

Getting a massage is very helpful to a pain patient in physical therapy. Massage increases blood flow to an injured area, relieving stiffness and swelling, relaxes tense muscles, and increases the levels of natural endorphins. There are many different kinds of massage, all of which are helpful in this primary stage of physical therapy. There is no single method that works better than another—it is simply a matter of what feels best to you. If one kind of massage is uncomfortable, try another kind, until you find one that is effective. This is not a mandatory element of Step Three but any therapy that involves human touch, whether it's from a massage therapist, a friend, or even yourself, usually makes a patient feel better. Before you turn your attention to this therapy, make sure your medication treatments are having an effect on your pain, and that you have started a stretch routine.

Each massage technique has a slightly different approach, so choose the ones that work best for you. When you seek out a massage therapist (and many physical therapists are trained in massage), ask your doctor or your friends whom they recommend. Here are some varieties of massage therapy:

• Standard "Swedish" muscle-kneading massage, developed by a nineteenth-century Swedish gymnast named Per Henrik Ling. His theory was that massage was a sort of "passive" gymnastic exercise to help heal and tone muscles.

- Shiatsu, a Japanese massage that uses finger pressure along the same meridians as acupuncture does. In the Far East, this type of massage is believed to be more beneficial in the long run, as opposed to traditional Western massage such as Swedish massage.
- Rolfing is very intense pressure and manipulation of deep muscle and tissue with the hands, named for the woman who innovated this technique, a biophysicist named Ida Rolf.
- Reflexology—As with acupuncture, the Chinese identified deep thumb pressure on key spots of the foot as effective with various organs throughout the body. Some patients like this massage simply because they like having their feet rubbed.

You might also rely on the healing hands of your partner or loved one. Even a nonprofessional massage can clear your mind, improve your mood, and stimulate relaxing energy. Advise your therapist if you are pregnant or have any injuries or pain. Scented oils add to the relaxing atmosphere, and aim for at least forty-five minutes to achieve maximum effects of massage. Many types of electrical at-home massage units have been found very helpful, particularly for cancer patients.

Ultrasound

Ultrasound treatment is a method of deep massage that increases blood flow to all the structures deep within the body, beyond the reach of normal manual massage. The ultrasound machine uses sound waves to warm muscles up to four centimeters below the skin. It also helps with surface muscles, but it is particularly helpful in pain areas that are hard to reach because they are too deep. These devices can be found at most rehabilitation centers, and your physical therapist can show you how they work. It is an effective therapy for all types of pain.

TENS

TENS, or transcutaneous electrical nerve stimulation, forces a muscle spasm to relax by overstimulating it with mild electrical impulses. It might sound strange, to break a spasm by creating another kind of spasm, but it's one way to fatigue muscles that are out of control. A TENS unit is a small battery-operated unit, about the size of a Walkman, with up to eight electrodes that are applied to the skin near the pain. The electrodes are strategically placed to surround the pain area and to stimulate it from every direction. The TENS unit sends an electric current through the skin and into the muscle. This "counter-irritant" is painless, but it causes so many messages to travel from the muscle to the brain that the brain stops feeling pain and only feels the benign electric stimulation. This technique is also believed to increase the body's levels of endorphins. The TENS unit has controls for intensity, speed, and depth of stimulation, so the patient can adjust it to reach his or her own pain-relieving levels. There are no side effects from this pain relief technique, and it can be safely used for a wide variety of pain symptoms. TENS is good to use in conjunction with other therapies, because it attacks your pain from yet another angle. Your doctor can provide you with the TENS device and can show you how to use it on your own, whenever you feel you need it. For roughly 70 percent of pain patients, TENS is very effective on muscle spasms, certain post-op pain, and nerve pain. Talk to your pain doctor or physical therapist about how TENS might help your recovery.

Chiropractic

This discipline essentially relates the position of the vertebrae to a healthy nervous system. Even a small misalignment in the spine can cause a nerve pain as well as chronic muscle spasm as an involuntary reflex. Finding this misalignment and adjusting the vertebrae to their normal positions can be very helpful in breaking the spasm and regaining flexibility. Chiropractic care can help "reset" the area of discomfort and unblock painful nerve pathways. This is not a necessity for the Painbuster program, unless it is part of your physical therapy regimen. I have seen pain patients who were greatly helped by chiropractors. However, many patients make the mistake of relying solely on chiropractors. This might relieve pain for a temporary period, but until your pain is attacked by the entire arsenal in this program, it will keep returning. Patrick E. had lower back pain, and he was much improved after eight weekly visits to a chiropractor. One year later, however, the pain returned, only it was much worse. He had been compensating for what had been a herniated disc, and now the entire dynamics in his spine had been altered by bad muscle memory. This caused new muscular pain, which, in turn, aggravated the herniated disc. The additional pressure on his sciatic nerve required immediate disc surgery to prevent permanent nerve damage. Chiropractic treatment itself is not harmful, but postponing proper treatment can be. A chiropractor can help you feel better, but I recommend this treatment as one part of a wider physical therapy program. Be sure you see a doctor in addition to a chiropractor.

Go Slowly

More time and focus must be devoted to this beginning stage than to any other part of physical therapy. Flexibility and function are the foundation for all subsequent rehabilitation for the pain patient. Getting the stretches and alignment correct takes more care than the other exercises. But it is imperative to complete this stage properly—under supervision of a physical therapist—before moving on.

STRENGTHENING

After flexibility and function are restored, the muscles must be strengthened to maintain progress and to prevent future injury. Despite its name, the goal of this stage is not necessarily to add extra muscle strength like a weight lifter, but to restore basic muscle tone. Strengthening allows you to handle simple daily tasks such as walking to work or sweeping the floor. This goal varies widely from one person to the next: a seventy-year-old grandmother has a far different lifestyle than a twenty-year-old athlete, so her goals must be adjusted accordingly.

Strengthening muscles actually has several benefits. When muscles are used, their tendons—the tissues that attach muscles to bones—are also becoming stronger. With increased activity, there is more blood flow to the whole area, offering extra nourishment to muscles while carrying away large amounts of lactic acid. Although we're not muscle-building for super biceps and deltoids, strengthening will add a little bulk to the "bellies" of all muscles. Bulkier muscles take stress off the bones in a joint. Imagine your muscles as a rubber band: a thick rubber band can handle a lot more pressure than a thin one. A thick muscle offers more support to a joint than a thin muscle. The renewed bulk also reduces the chance of a muscle spasm and naturally limits the motion of a joint, such as an elbow or knee, so it won't overextend itself.

Strength is important to body function, but if the function is not corrected first, the strength can cause more problems instead. Muscle groups that are being properly strengthened are also having their mirror-opposite muscle groups strengthened. The opposing muscles on each side need equal strength to prevent an imbalance or injury. If you begin strengthening exercises without having restored flexibility and function, your opposing muscles may not develop at the same rate. In fact, without restoring normal function first, opposing muscle groups can move farther apart in strength, rather than together. If you continue to "favor" an aching shoulder, the mirror-opposite shoulder muscles will gain more strength than the ailing one. This defeats the purpose of strengthening, and this is why you should always restore flexibility and function before moving on to strengthening routines. Also, all muscles are anchored by tendons—if one muscle pulls harder than the other, then it's possible for it to pull away the opposing tendon from its anchor. As a patient exercises both sets of opposing muscles, the tendons are being strengthened so they can handle more pressure, too.

When you lift something heavy out of the trunk of a car, you are demanding the lower back do something it was not meant to do: to twist and lift at the same time. If the muscles—and the tendons—are strong in the lower back, then the exertion will be solid and stable. There is small likelihood of injury. Not only that, but the strong muscles surrounding the spine contribute to the size of the entire joint—in this case, the spine—and transfers much of the joint pressure onto muscles instead of discs and bones. You can really tell the difference in the lower back area. When those muscles are in good shape, they are virtual shock absorbers. If you have recovered from a herniated disc and you've strengthened the lower back muscles with physical therapy, the larger spine muscles even help each disc maintain its natural position in the vertebrae. These larger muscles give a little more room to a space that was being squeezed in the first place.

If the abdominal muscles are also strengthened, then they will better control the twisting motion, making it less likely for lifting something out of a car trunk to stress the lower back. Healthy abdominal muscles restrict the twist— we call this motion torque—as the strengthened lower back muscles absorb the weight. The spine doesn't have to do anything. Those healthy abs prevent torque motion in the spine, which cannot handle it. No one gets hurt.

Your exercise program should be easy to do and appropriate for all your muscle groups, not just the ones in your pain area. Here are some sample exercises that provide a well-rounded start to your strengthening routine. Be sure to review these with your physical therapist before doing them.

Standing Calf Lift

Targets the muscles in the calves.

1. Stand with your feet shoulder width apart and hold on to the top of a dresser, countertop, or the back of a chair, keeping your stomach tight and neck straight to maintain proper alignment. Inhale.
2. Slowly rise up onto your toes. Exhale. Hold the position for 5 to 10 seconds, breathing evenly. Return slowly to the starting position.

You may also lift and lower one foot at a time. (Simply keep the other heel slightly off the ground while doing the exercise.)

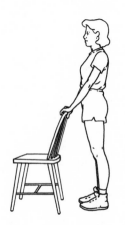 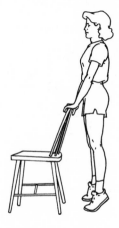

Sit-to-Standing Squat

Targets the muscles in the front of the thighs, hips, back, and abdomen.

1. Sit all the way back on a sturdy, armless chair with your shoulders down and relaxed (the back of the chair should be straight and positioned near a wall, if possible). Keep your stomach in, chin tucked, gaze forward, and head upright. Inhale.

2. Stand, lifting your body about ⅔ of the way up. Keep your back straight, stomach tight, neck straight, and knees slightly bent (be sure your knee joints are slightly behind or just over your ankle joints). Exhale as you lift your body. Hold the position for 5 to 10 seconds, breathing evenly. Return slowly to the starting position.

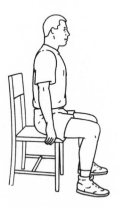 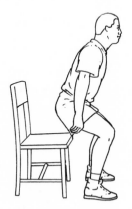

Abdominal Bridge

Targets the muscles in the buttocks, thighs, abdomen, and back.

1. Lie on your back with your knees bent and your feet flat on the floor. Keep your stomach tight, your neck straight, and the small of your back pressed toward the floor to maintain proper alignment. Keep your arms at your sides, palms down. Inhale.

2. Keeping your stomach tight, perform a bridging movement by pinching your buttocks together as you lift them off the floor. Exhale as you lift your buttocks. Hold the position for 5 to 10 seconds, breathing evenly. Return slowly to the starting position.

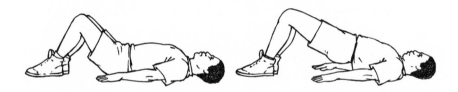

Kickback

Targets the muscles in the buttocks, back, and upper thighs.

Note: *This exercise can be done with light ankle weights.*

1. Kneel down on your hands and knees. Keep your stomach in, chin tucked, gaze downward, and head and neck in alignment. Inhale.

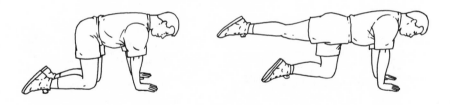

2. Slowly lift one leg out in the air, keeping your knee as straight as possible so your thigh is level with your body. Exhale as you lift your leg. Hold the position for 5 to 10 seconds, breathing evenly. *Do not hold the position if using weights.* Return slowly to the starting position.

3. Repeat on the opposite side.

Abdominal Crunch with Arms at Sides

Targets the muscles in the abdomen.

1. Lie on your back with your knees bent and your feet flat on the floor. Keep your stomach tight, your neck straight, and the small of your back pressed toward the floor to maintain proper alignment. Keep your arms at your sides, palms down. Inhale.

2. With your stomach tight and chin tucked, slowly lift just your head and shoulders up, keeping your arms next to your sides (not down on the floor), until the upper part of your shoulder blades lifts off the floor. (Do not use your arms to push yourself up.) Exhale as you lift. Hold the position for 5 to 10 seconds, breathing evenly. Return slowly to the starting position.

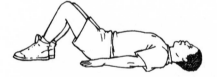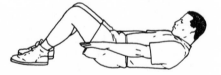

Abdominal Crunch with Crossed Arms

Targets the muscles in the abdomen and the front of the neck.

1. Lie on your back with your knees bent and your feet flat on the floor. Keep your stomach tight, your neck straight, and the small of your back pressed toward the floor to maintain proper alignment. Cross your arms over your chest. Inhale.

2. With your stomach tight and chin tucked, slowly lift just your head and shoulders up until the upper part of your shoulder blades lifts off the floor. Exhale as you lift. Hold the position for 5 to 10 seconds, breathing evenly. Return slowly to the starting position.

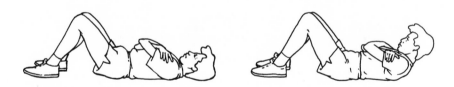

Side Arm Lift

Targets the muscles in the shoulders and upper back.

Note: *This exercise uses hand weights.*

1. Sit all the way back on a sturdy, armless chair, feet up on a small footstool, with your shoulders down and relaxed (the back of the chair should be straight and positioned near a wall, if possible). Keep your stomach

in, chin tucked, gaze forward, and head upright. The weights should be down at your sides, with your palms facing inward, and your elbows slightly bent. Inhale.

2. Keeping your shoulders down, slowly lift both your arms out to the sides until the weights are as close to shoulder height as comfortable. Exhale as you lift your arms. Inhale as you return slowly to the starting position.

You may also lift and lower one arm at a time, or have your palms facing forward, with the thumbs pointed toward the ceiling, as you lift.

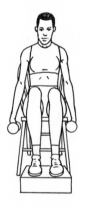
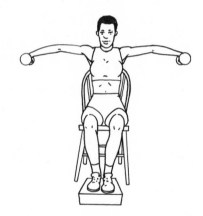

Biceps Curl

Targets the muscles in the front of the upper arms and wrists.

Note: *This exercise uses hand weights.*

1. Sit all the way back on a sturdy, armless chair, feet up on a small footstool, with your shoulders down and relaxed (the back of the chair should be

straight and positioned near a wall, if possible). Keep your stomach in, chin tucked, gaze forward, and head upright. The weights should be down at your sides, with your palms facing forward, and your elbows straight but soft. Inhale.

2. Slowly bend your elbows and bring the weights up to a 90-degree angle. Exhale as you lift your arms. Inhale as you return slowly to the starting position.

You may also lift and lower one arm at a time.

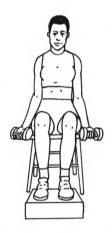 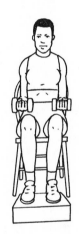

CONDITIONING

Conditioning is the phase that widens your exercise routine to include the entire body. There is actually a limit to how much you can work on one part of the body to the exclusion of everything else. As rehabilitation progresses, you should already start seeing improvements all over, for your body is indeed returning to good condition. As you improve, the cardiovascular system is increasing its ability to handle exercise, so there should now be more body parts involved. As time passes, the exercise should become aerobic, which essentially means it should make you short of breath and make your heart beat faster. Walking, swimming, jogging, bicycling, stair climbing, rowing, video aerobics classes, Tae-Bo, and step workouts are just a few activities that can get your body moving into condition. I am a huge proponent of walking. It is easy, accessible, inexpensive, and one of the most enjoyable exercises you can do. Work your way up to a twenty-minute brisk walk, at least every other day, and you will find yourself feeling better and sleeping better, too.

There is less need for a physical therapist during the conditioning phase, although one can still provide assistance and support. You should prepare to take everything you have learned from physical therapy and apply it to your entire lifestyle. Conditioning exercises should be done at least three days a week, for at least twenty minutes at a time. Always warm up before and cool down after. This means do the activity very slowly during the first five minutes, and slowly again during the last five minutes.

Perhaps you're saying to yourself, well, this all sounds great, but how do I find a place that will help me with a program like this? Using the information you now have about flexibility and function, strengthening, and conditioning, telephone or visit some physical therapy centers (some resources are listed at the end of this book). Ask therapists about the three stages of physical therapy. They should be familiar with them, as well as other aspects of pain rehabilitation. Ask them which of your muscle groups should be worked on during recovery from your particular pain syndrome. In addition, a good book containing hun-

Walking is one of the best exercises a pain patient can do on a regular basis, but I believe that nothing is more effective than exercising in water. Moving under water can be better than moving in air, particularly if the temperature of the water is heated to help increase blood flow to the muscles. Heat makes all exercise more tolerable to your muscles. In addition, there is far less stress on your joints when they are underwater than when they are working on dry land. Water buoys a patient's entire body weight, making it easier to exercise without every last pound bearing down on the injured area. Someone with a replaced hip joint, for example, can walk on an underwater treadmill with greater ease than he can walk on a regular treadmill. Because of the low joint pressure of an underwater workout, this patient can even begin rehabilitation earlier, and be healed more quickly. The same goals can be reached without underwater therapy but, as you can see, there are advantages to at least starting out with aquatic exercises.

dreds of physical therapy exercises is the *American Physical Therapy Association Guide to Physical Therapy* (published by Holt, and available at most book retailers), which might also offer guidelines to help in your program.

It is crucial that the three stages of physical therapy be performed correctly, and that means while pain is absent. Be patient. If you are still in pain, do not begin any physical therapy. It will not help you if the pain is still there. If doing any exercise causes pain, stop doing it and consult your doctor or therapist.

Physical therapy can seem boring and tedious, but no new technology or medication can replace it. Odd as it may seem, since it is so "low-tech," the benefits of physical therapy were only discovered in the last few decades. Only after researchers started documenting patients' progress did they see how effective physical therapy was in healing chronic pain. Pain-relieving medications may have helped us get to this point, but pain-management specialists know that the human body was indeed designed to heal itself.

CHAPTER 6

Customize a Maintenance Program That Works: Diet, Stress Control, Emotional Support, and Exercise

Step Four: Pain-Free for Life

The last step is the most important one of the Pain-buster program. The body has been carefully taken through three steps to return to a normal healthy state. Now you must take one final step to ensure that the pain doesn't come back. This step includes many options, some of which may not be necessary for your case. The goal is to choose the combination of elements that you can stick with and rotate—the ones that work to keep your pain away. All patients must complete this step to succeed with the Pain-buster program. If certain modifications in your lifestyle aren't made after the pain syndrome is corrected or if proper maintenance is ignored, the problem will return.

Think of all the people you know who have struggled through weight-loss diets. After several months, when they've finally reached their goal, they look terrific. So they stop dieting. They haven't set up a careful maintenance program—a readjusted diet and exercise routine—

either because they don't know how to, or they think it's not necessary since the weight is gone already. Over the course of a few weeks, they then gain back all the weight they'd lost. This is a very common scenario. It is not unlike what can happen with a pain syndrome. After all, whatever the cause, there was a reason for the chronic pain to occur in the first place. Even though we may have removed the pain and rehabilitated the body, we have to map out a continued plan to permanently obliterate its cause and to prevent the return of pain.

This is not only the most important step in the Painbuster program, it is also the most difficult. You don't immediately see the benefits of doing this step. Motivation is never easy. It's like saving for retirement. You know you should do it, but there won't be any immediate repercussion if it's not at the top of your list. This step does not require you to join aerobics classes or to start weight lifting with a personal trainer. The Painbuster program is flexible enough to work for the laziest and most sedentary of patients. You will have to do more than just read this book. But this step requires much less effort than if you were still trying to conduct your daily life with chronic pain.

Once you become an exerciser, your entire lifestyle changes. You start to feel good, so you start to eat better to enhance that feeling, and you become more and more fit and healthy. It is an empowering feeling, and one that makes most people feel very satisfied, healthy, and happy. It is remarkable to see the transformation in someone who begins even a very modest exercise routine.

The maintenance program varies according to your condition, but it consists primarily of two or more of these elements:

- increasing and maintaining muscle tone
- diet modification
- continued medication management
- stress reduction counseling

MUSCLE TONE

Hefty muscles are not the goal here. Muscle bulk is not as important as maintaining a balance of normal strength and flexibility. Increasing muscle tone and maintaining muscle mass simply mean finding conditioning activities—walking, swimming, biking, and so forth—that you will continue to do on a fairly regular basis, at least three times a week for twenty minutes or more. Many people are very busy, and it can be a challenge to find an activity that will consistently draw them away from everything else.

It's helpful to understand from the outset that your activity might rotate or change with the seasons. You might get bored with just one activity. Look at it as an opportunity to design an exercise rotation you enjoy, which includes periodically moving on to something new. Go ahead and buy the cross-country ski machine. You will use it for a while, and then you might tire of it. This is fine, as long as you move on to something else. Don't feel guilty if you never use the ski machine again, and don't anticipate that this "failure" precludes your need to start a new activity. Give the old machine to a friend. But you must pick up another activity in its place.

Sixty-year-old Florence S. had chronic pain from a herniated disc. We soothed the large nerve irritation with a series of three epidural steroid injections, along with a combination of Motrin and Zoloft. In physical therapy, we strengthened her lower back and abdomen to empower her against further twisting injuries. She was fine for about eight months. When winter came, Florence lost interest in her daily one-mile walk because it was too cold outside. Rather than planning a replacement indoor activity, she simply let her exercise lapse. After only two months of inactivity, she lost muscle tone, flexibility, and soon strained her lower back with a small injury that normally wouldn't have hurt anyone. It had been easy for Florence to measure her progress during the first three steps of the Painbuster program. But the fourth one—maintaining her good health and pain-free life—was easy to take for granted and she let it lapse. It wasn't long before Florence's pain syndrome revived, and she had to start over at Step One.

Because you have to rely on yourself for motivation, make it as easy for yourself as possible. It helps if you enjoy the activity, or if you have a friend to keep you company. Any aerobic activity—one that gets your heart beating faster and your lungs working—will keep your muscles toned, your arteries clear, and it will increase your body's regular production of endorphins, the natural pain reliever. People who don't exercise have a lower tolerance for pain, and their weak muscles are more likely to tense and spasm. This fourth step simply makes you more resistant to all pain.

A regular activity of at least one hundred minutes per week also raises your basal metabolic rate (BMR). This is your body's natural estimate of how much energy it burns on a daily basis. As you exercise more, perhaps twenty minutes a day, your body will burn more fat on a regular basis, and its basal metabolic rate will increase. Once the BMR is at a higher level, it will stay at that higher fat-burning rate for some time, *even on days when you don't work out at all.* The more you exercise on a regular basis, the higher your BMR will become over the course of several months. Your body will then simply burn more calories during all hours of the day and night.

Muscle tone can be maintained any number of ways—going to the gym, swimming, walking, working the rowing machines, using treadmills, stair climbing, bicycling, and participating in organized activities such as dancing, step classes, karate, or Tae-Bo. Any single one of these, or any combination of them, three or four times a week, is enough to maintain good muscle tone forever. When your energy is flagging, tell yourself to give it five minutes. Tell yourself you can stop after five minutes. You are in control! Very often, five minutes of exercise will motivate you to continue for a few more. If not, that's okay. Save it for another day. Just try to get to one hundred minutes a week. Be careful to spend the first five minutes doing the exercise slowly, in order to warm up. Then conclude your exercise by doing it slowly for another five minutes at the end, to cool down.

I highly recommend that you show all activities to a physical therapist, to ensure that they are being properly done. Consult your physical therapist, or even a certified trainer at your local recreation center or health club. It's a good idea to return to this trainer once in a while, perhaps every other month, to demonstrate your current exercise, and to learn how to do it correctly before you do it for too long. Without supervision, poorly performed exercises can develop into a bad habit that could injure you. By getting a physical therapist to evaluate your exercise program from time to time, you can be confident that it is helping you maintain good muscle tone.

DIET

Almost every health condition is affected by a person's diet. Diabetes, hypertension, chronic pancreatitis, and gall-bladder disease, just to name a few, are diseases that demand close attention to what you eat. Most people don't eat perfectly all the time. They fast, then binge on bad foods, or simply don't pay attention and put practically anything into their mouths. As with exercise, our diets are largely limited by our busy lifestyles: no breakfast, fast-food lunch, take-out dinner, snacks on the run.

There is no magic diet that will prevent all pain syndromes. Nor is there a single food (or lack thereof) that causes pain. Some people think one or more of the following foods, however, can make pain syndromes worse:

- dairy products
- eggs
- wheat and wheat flour
- tomatoes
- meat
- citrus fruits
- corn
- eggplant

I believe such intolerance depends on the individual and may be caused by food allergies that exacerbate the pain syndrome, rather than by food directly "causing" pain. By eliminating each of these foods, one at a time, you might learn whether your body has a negative reaction to them.

At the other end of this spectrum, here are some foods that are said to *fight* pain:

- fresh ginger
- garlic
- foods containing vitamin B_6, such as broccoli, beans, potatoes, and spinach
- cold-water fish, such as tuna, halibut, squid, swordfish, salmon, mackerel, cod, herring, and rainbow trout, all of which contain omega-3 and essential unsaturated fatty acids.

I suspect that these healthy foods are not specifically pain fighters, but are great sources of energy that support muscle tone. Decreasing body fat is a good goal for any diet, particularly for pain syndromes involving the lower back. The lower back carries much of your extra weight, and it is also the place that must adjust your body's center of balance to accommodate extra weight. If you gain weight, in other words, your lower back carries all the extra pounds, no matter where they are.

I think a connection between low-fat diets and good back health has been established. A low-fat diet is common among Japanese-American women, and studies have shown that they have *half* the risk of back pain that other American women do. Among many other studies, this one illustrates that more back pain patients should consider a diet rich in grains, vegetables, and beans. And, of course, you should always drink plenty of water so that all of your body's systems function normally and without stress.

There are several books on low-fat diets for lifetime health maintenance that I recommend to pain patients, including *Dr. Dean Ornish's Program for Reversing Heart Disease*, Dr. Neal Barnard's *Food for Life*, and Dr. Andrew Weil's *Eight Weeks to Optimal Health*. You can design your own low-fat diet, however, so that it keeps you satisfied and energized. Here are some good tips to help establish your personal diet guidelines:

  · Eat fewer calories by cutting the amount of fat you consume. Limit your consumption of meat, cheese, whole milk, cream, and butter. However, try to make your calories as tasty as possible so that you feel satisfied. Sometimes it's better to eat toast with real butter than with margarine, or regular cookies instead of low-fat snacks, because you might feel more sated by the lower amounts of "real thing" than by greater volumes of "healthy substitutes."

- Use only olive, canola, peanut, or avocado oil in your cooking. Avoid vegetable shortening and poly-unsaturated vegetable oils such as corn, sesame, sun-flower, and safflower oils.
- Eat protein in the form of grains (whole grains, please!), beans, eggs, soy, nuts, and small amounts of lean meat.
- Eat plenty of fruits and vegetables every day.
- Drink lots of water.

If you put even a little effort into monitoring your food intake, you will succeed in maintaining a pain-free life. Good nutrition won't necessarily eliminate pain by itself, but it helps to relieve stress on your body and boosts your immune system and general good health.

CONTINUED MEDICATION

The long-term success of the Painbuster program frequently requires the use of oral medications, even after the physical therapy is complete and the pain is resolved. In most Painbuster cases, the drugs are used temporarily to reduce pain while the body repairs the damage. This might take several months, or it could take a couple of years. Medications such as tricyclic antidepressants often take several weeks to build up to their maximum thera-peutic effects anyway, accumulating slowly to reach total pain relief. Once that level has been reached, then we maintain the medications to ensure the condition is properly treated. After the pain has been resolved, we recommend keeping the medication regimen for two or three months afterward, and then tapering off very slowly. If the pain begins to return while tapering the medications, then we will keep the medications full strength until pain relief is maintained for several months.

Some people believe that if they are feeling better, they can stop taking the medications. It is usually a mistake to discontinue the medications the moment you have returned to good health. If medication resolved a muscle spasm, then stopping it will probably return the muscle to its "memory" of a spasm state. *Maintain medications until the original pain syndrome has been gone for several months.* Otherwise there is a risk that the pain will return. With most conditions, we start with higher doses of the appropriate medications and, when the desired effect has been achieved, we taper them off slightly. We want to use the minimal amount possible, but we want to keep the condition under control. When this minimal amount is determined, it is continued until several months after the pain is gone.

Sometimes a pain syndrome is only controlled as long as the medications continue. In other words, there are cases where medication remains part of the regular maintenance program. This is still not the permanent cure. Even continued medications are used primarily to enable the patient to keep exercising and to maintain functional life. It is preferable to stopping the medications and subsequently stopping the exercise and proper diet. The work you do while on medications will perpetuate the good health you have reached through physical therapy. I have one patient who still takes Elavil after seven pain-free years, and another patient with diabetes who needs a regular dose of Mexitil to keep pain away. They continue to exercise and eat right, and they continue to take safe medications that keep them pain-free.

Sometimes the body gets so accustomed to a particular medication that the drug loses its effectiveness. We then rotate to another similar medication, in order to maintain pain relief. If you sense that your medication is no longer as helpful as it once was, then you might consider moving on to a new one. Almost every medication class has several different options. Even an over-the-counter nonsteroidal anti-inflammatory should be rotated every month. Start with Advil, then move on to Aleve, then to Orudis, and so forth. You have more than twenty to choose from, and each works in a slightly different way. Keep a list of the ones that work and the ones that don't. Discuss them with your doctor. Using trial and error and rotating through the ones that work are important for long-term care when your pain condition demands medication maintenance.

STRESS REDUCTION

One of the most common underlying causes of pain is stress. Most of us are familiar with stress to some degree. It is the "fight or flight" biological instinct for our bodies to tense muscles and adjust blood flow during moments of stress. This is a proven fact. When people speak of "internalizing" a problem, they may not realize how true this is.

Stress can be particularly taxing on the back muscles, and I believe it is the reason why lower back pain is the dominant syndrome of all my patients. Returning a newly pain-free patient to his old life of stress is a guarantee that I'll be seeing him again before long. To remain pain-free, this patient must learn new ways to cope with stress, to "externalize" stress in a helpful way, and to give his poor muscles a break. This can also help the rest of his family as well, since the chronic pain of one member often affects the emotional well-being of the entire household. I once had a patient, Walter S., a forty-six-year-old television executive who had suffered from a herniated disc pain for years. As he progressed through this final step of stress reduction, I was pleased to note that his wife's hay fever "magically" disappeared for good, and he started coaching softball for his teenage daughter's team.

I do not think there is a single pain syndrome that can be treated solely with stress management. However, too many times, a patient's pain is approached only from a psychological angle, without regard to the real physical cause of the pain. This is wrong. I believe it is one reason why patients get the notion that their pain is all in their heads. They may even do things to prove it is not imaginary pain—such as subconsciously cause themselves to be injured. These patients also become very defensive and work against their baffled health-care providers. Stress makes all pain syndromes worse, and all pain syndromes create some degree of stress. Even if there are psychological causes, your pain is real and must be treated like any other pain.

It is important to identify what is causing your stress and to eliminate this cause from your life. But more important, I believe in first removing the pain. After the pain is gone, then perhaps you and your doctor can determine the psychological components that remain. But as long as the pain is there, it's going to be very difficult to pinpoint the stress triggers behind the physical pain.

Muscle spasm is the type of pain most commonly associated with stress, because the transmitters of stress are the same neurotransmitters of muscle spasms. Pain conditions that include muscle spasms respond very well to stress counseling, but only after the actual spasm has been treated first and the pain is gone. After the pain is eliminated, in most cases, the psychological elements—and the stress—become much reduced anyway. They are no longer being fed by the pain.

Stress reduction can take many forms in pain management. One-on-one sessions with a therapist can help a patient cope with a chronic disease. This requires a commitment from the patient, in terms of time and money, but private counseling can be the quickest and most effective way, because all the attention is focused on your stress. In certain cases, the underlying cause of pain might be a hidden memory or a foundering relationship that is not yet resolved. Another good option is to attend a group therapy session, in addition to, or instead of, private counseling. Group sessions with patients who have similar problems can help participants use their common issues to support one another. They also allow people to observe other pain patients who are at different stages of recovery and to gauge their own progress. Group sessions are very popular, because information about individual pain syndromes is shared quickly, giving other patients resources—in the form of other patients—of support. Also, group sessions are less expensive, which is important since most health-care plans do not cover psychological counseling for chronic pain management. I have one group of various sales reps who call themselves the Stress Force and another group of HIV patients who meet at the local coffee shop once a week. Of course, new friendships with people who understand your condition don't cost you a dime.

The goal is to allow you to identify the causes of your stress, and then to find a way to control them so that normal life is not disrupted. Stress reduction is best maintained while continuing physical therapy and medication management, so that all facets of pain relief are being used at once. Stress counseling need not be long-term, but during the final stages of this program it can help close the door forever on an old pain problem. Sometimes, in rare cases, stress management even involves changing your job or your living situation. Counseling will help you make these seemingly impossible changes, so that you can live without chronic pain.

Relaxation techniques such as meditation and yoga provide patients with stress control that they can implement on their own. They are most helpful when used in combination with stress group sessions or private counseling. Relaxation techniques frequently help a patient regain control over the issues in her life. This is obviously a personal choice, depending on what you are comfortable doing.

Biofeedback is a technique that enables a patient to measure the level of tension he is feeling, as well as the level of relaxation. This device has noninvasive sticky electrodes (not the needles for the more precise EMG diagnostic test) and an electronic measuring scale that the patient uses to rate one muscle group at a time. Patients can experiment with relaxation techniques of any kind, and periodically use a biofeedback device to confirm how effective the methods are. Some patients can see on a biofeedback computer screen, for example, if their muscles are really relaxed after doing yoga. If not, that patient might move on to meditation instead and use biofeedback to gauge that method's impact on his body. Biofeedback helps you control pain by making you aware of subtle changes in your body and how to move your body in healthy ways. This technique can be particularly helpful for patients with chronic muscle spasms or fibromyalgia.

Here are some relaxation and meditation techniques that might help you. Try practicing one of these every day for a week and see what effect it can have on your stress levels.

Sit in a chair, or sit or lie down on the floor, in a comfortable position. Close your eyes and listen to your natural breathing. Follow the flow as you breathe in, and relax your chest muscles as you breathe out. Focus your thoughts on your breath, even if it changes slightly. Every time you breathe out, try to exhale more air than you took in. You can control the intercostal rib muscles used for exhalation, and every time you breathe out more, you will automatically inhale more. Continue this for at least five minutes.

After a few days, work your way up to ten minutes. Most people take sixteen breaths per minute. See if you can work your way to four breaths a minute. Think of nothing except your breathing, exhaling slowly and deeply, and letting the inhale increase on its own. Try to do this every day.

Find a quiet place to sit comfortably. Relax all your muscles, beginning with your face and neck, then down to your shoulders and back, hips and legs. Find one thought or prayer, a small mental device that you find soothing, and focus on this thought for ten minutes. Set a timer if it helps you to stop monitoring a clock. If intrusive thoughts enter your mind, don't embrace them or follow them—just let them go and return to your "mantra." For some people, it helps to listen to a musical chant. Do this for ten or fifteen minutes every day.

Other good activities to help relieve stress:

- Go out for a vigorous walk, wherever you are. Breathe deeply and force negative thoughts from your mind by picking up the pace. Promise yourself just five minutes but try for twenty.
- Add music to the air to clear stressful thoughts from your mind. Crashing rock and roll, favorite oldies, or spiritual chants can alter your mood significantly.
- Take a bath, and make a ritual of it. Add scented bath oils or lighted candles, and don't let anyone disturb you for twenty minutes. Play soft music, close your eyes, and take slow, deep breaths.
- Do the crossword puzzle, cook, knit, read, play cards, bounce a basketball—find any activity that can take your mind away from the moment. Your thoughts deserve a break on a frequent basis.

With patients who have a great deal of psychological elements triggering their pain syndromes, one of the greatest challenges is getting them to acknowledge that a psychological aspect even exists. In other words, the patients who need stress reduction most are the ones who will usually deny that stress is a factor. Perhaps they fear that their pain may not be treated medically if they admit that psychological forces might be involved. These people might think that their pain will be treated as though it were imaginary pain. I have found that using biofeedback techniques can help these patients see the benefits of stress counseling. Overlapping counseling with other maintenance options is very helpful and, in many cases, the pain will not go away until the psychological issues are addressed. At the least, stress counseling makes it more likely that you will be permanently and completely cured.

Pain centers offer group sessions for stress reduction, as well as private counseling, although this is not a program prerequisite such as physical therapy. But when my patients see the scientific evidence connecting stress with chronic pain, they usually want to try at least one group session. They're pleased to discover that stress counseling not only helps control pain, but it improves their lives in other ways as well.

While some patients have a sense of rebirth after the pain is gone, other people have difficulty adjusting to a life without pain, particularly if the pain syndrome was a prevalent aspect of their lives. Others have learned to enjoy life most fully when there is a little pain in the background. As part of the maintenance program, I support whatever makes the patient comfortable, even if it means keeping a little pain. If patients are happy and they can function normally, who are we to say they shouldn't feel the way they choose? Pain is a very personal thing.

Pain-Proof Your Home and Office

"An extra firm mattress with our coil-spring technology will cure your bad back!" If what some ads claimed were true, my waiting room would be empty. Many people believe that the density of a mattress improves sleep and good spine health. I happen to believe there is no difference between a soft mattress and a hard mattress—you should choose whichever you prefer.

Far more important, in my estimation, is the ergonomics of your workplace. You spend more time there than in your bed anyway. I'll bet that you have not examined how you use your desk, chair, phone, keyboard, and computer monitor. The next time you sit down at your workstation, look around and consider these factors for proper ergonomics:

Chair: Your most important piece of office furniture is the one on which you sit. Even with a limited budget or resources, spend a little time and effort to get a good office chair. The best type is a chair with armrests that adjust and rise to your elbows. It should also offer good lumbar support, pressing your lower back into a natural, upright position. A chair with an adjustable seat height lets you set it so that your feet rest flat on the floor, with your knees bent at a comfortable ninety-degree angle. It helps if the chair swivels from side to side, but it is not essential to have it lean back or rock. My favorite office chair is manufactured by Steelcase, although there are many good options available at discount office supply stores.

If you work behind the steering wheel of a truck or car, try to approximate the driver's seat to the position of an armchair with elbow rests. Lumbar support can be in the form of a pillow, to keep your spine as comfortable and straight as possible. Wherever you work, taking frequent breaks from a constant sitting or standing position is essential. Once per hour, try to do some stretching exercises.

Desk and/or Keyboard: Your work surface should be an inch or two lower than your elbows when you're seated in your desk chair. This is usually lower than most people think is correct. Having your elbows bent no more than ninety degrees means your wrists will be straight, most of the time. If necessary, your wrists will be more likely to lean down than to bend up, if your work surface is lower than your elbows. This is the most ergonomic way to help prevent the onset of carpal tunnel syndrome. If your desk is too high and you can't change it, then raise your seat level and rest your feet on a box. Keep your elbows on your armrests and prop your wrists, if necessary, to keep them straight while you do the bulk of your tasks.

Monitor: The top of your computer monitor should be two to six inches below your eye level when you're at your workstation. To keep your eyes looking up will cause eyestrain and, perhaps, a headache or neck pain. Even if your screen is perfectly level with your eyes, your head tends to lean down toward your work surface, forcing your eyes to look up. Lower the monitor, take it off the hard drive, or even move it from the desk surface, whatever it takes to get it slightly lower than your eye level. Don't put it so low, however, that you strain your neck downward.

Telephone: Every time you hold a phone receiver up to your ear, your body is in an unnatural position. If you work a lot on the phone, try to get a headset instead of using a normal receiver. This will remove regular crimping of your neck, shoulder, and elbow. Headsets are widely available and quite inexpensive, and most can adapt to any type of telephone.

Overlapping Is Key

It is rare that a patient simply returns pain-free to the same life she had before the onset of chronic pain. The transformation of body condition brings a renewed appreciation of good health and a new awareness of the inner and external factors that often accompany chronic pain. Make a list of the maintenance options that help you. Should you get bored or forget what they are, refer to this chapter again. Remind yourself of the diet, exercise, medication, or stress reduction tools that now fill the space in your life that was once occupied by chronic pain.

I wrote this book to clarify the elements of a program that was not easy to describe in one word, let alone one sentence. When their friends ask my patients "How did you get rid of your bad back?" they find themselves describing the four steps of the Painbuster program and wishing it didn't require so much explanation. Of all the elements that overlap in the Painbuster program, not one of them can be singled out as a simple answer to this question. But now that the four steps are explained in this book, the one-word answer is here: "Painbuster."

CHAPTER 7

The A to Z of Chronic Pain Syndromes

P ain syndromes are easier to understand when they are broken down into the six types of pain, and when you understand what parts of the body must be treated in order to achieve permanent pain relief. In this section, I will help unlock the mysteries and untangle the most common chronic pain syndromes by their various pain types. It may enable you to put your symptoms together with a name, or to take your syndrome apart so you can seek the proper cure. These symptoms and conditions are here to help you understand your diagnosis. Your own symptoms might vary, but this guide encompasses the general nature of the most common pain conditions.

I also review here some of the initial medication therapies for these pain syndromes, although, as you now know, most pain syndromes are primarily healed through physical therapy in conjunction with medications. These details will get you started in the right direction. Consult your doctor about putting the multidisciplinary Painbuster program to work for you.

ABDOMINAL PAIN

Chronic abdominal pain can come from many sources—pressure on internal organs, general muscle spasms we call stomach cramps, residual pain from lower back, or nerve or pelvis injury. The nervous system that senses pain in the "gut" is not specific, so this pain is often difficult to pinpoint. It is usually a deep, aching pain that stays within the abdominal area. The patient cannot always point to its exact location because it is a diffuse pain.

The most common sources for chronic abdominal pain are pancreatitis (due to alcoholism or cancer), hepatitis, postsurgical scarring or bowel obstruction, decreased blood flow to the organs in the abdomen, gastrointestinal disorders, or peritonitis, which is an irritation of the intestinal lining. It is essential to get a complete examination of the abdomen to determine the exact cause of pain. Most abdominal problems are "reversible," or capable of being cured. Once the ailment is reversed, the pain goes away. In most abdominal cases, treating the underlying problem is the only way to eliminate the pain permanently. Therefore, rather than consulting a pain-management specialist, you might start with an exam by an internist, gynecologist, or gastroenterologist.

In any case, I recommend getting pain relief from that doctor while the problem is being treated. If pain persists, or the problem still cannot be determined, then a pain-management specialist who is familiar with nerve blocks would be very helpful. I recommend medication therapy in the form of neuropathic pain agents, such as tricyclic antidepressants and perhaps a long-acting narcotic. I would also recommend an injection targeting the celiac plexus, the sensory nerve cluster that services everything in the abdomen. This would block the nerves to the abdominal area, reducing pain. The patient should choose whichever technique is available and most comfortable for him or her.

I also find that abdominal pain cases respond well to combining medications with psychological counseling. In fact, with abdominal pain, psychological counseling is an even more effective adjunct than physical therapy. The primary cause can be deceptive, but it's important to find out what is really behind this abdominal pain. Abdominal pain cases are frequently manifested by another chronic problem, such as a dysfunctional personal relationship, stress, a "nervous stomach," or poor diet.

See also Pelvic Pain.

ANKYLOSING SPONDYLITIS

This is an autoimmune disorder that falls under the large category of arthritis, and it seems to be hereditary. Anky-losing (stiffening) spondylitis (inflammation of the verte-brae) strikes primarily the sacroiliac joints that connect the pelvis to the spine. This disease damages the lower verte-brae until they become stiff and even fused together. The cause of ankylosing spondylitis is not known, and it usu-ally occurs in men over sixty years of age. It is progres-sively degenerative. It might start as a pain or stiffness in the lower back. The stiffness might then spread down the legs, mimicking the pain of sciatica. The pain may spread further, up the back and around the chest wall, sometimes even feeling like angina.

A simple blood test can confirm the presence of this disease. The treatments are identical to other arthritis remedies, such as medication combinations using nonsteroidal anti-inflammatories to reduce swelling. Physical therapy is also helpful, not only for pain relief, but in protecting against curvature of the spine. Regular exams and rotation of medications can control the pain of this disease, for which I highly recommend the array of treatments available through a pain-management specialist.

ARTHRITIS

More than forty million Americans suffer from arthritis. There are more than one hundred variations of this disease, and the most common form is osteoarthritis, where the cartilage degenerates and allows bones to rub together in the joints. This is a painful condition that limits movement and, up until recently, was primarily treated with acetaminophen (Tylenol) or nonsteroidal anti-inflammatory medications (such as Motrin or Advil), in spite of their irritating side effects. In recent years, arthritis sufferers have been much relieved by the compound known as glucosamine chondroitin sulfate. This natural substance is derived from shellfish and is now available in supermarkets and grocery stores. It gives you the building blocks and proper enzymes to build new cartilage, precluding the need for painkillers.

I have seen glucosamine chondroitin sulfates work miracles on pain patients who had been crippled by arthritis, and I highly recommend this compound. In addition to building cartilage with glucosamine chondroitin, the best defense against the pain of arthritis is physical therapy. I also recommend *The Arthritis Cure*, a comprehensive self-care guide by Dr. Jason Theodosakis, Brenda Adderly, and Barry Fox.

Rheumatoid arthritis is a different ailment completely; it is a disease of the immune system, and it can lead to overall weakness, fatigue, fever, and inflammation of the joints. Nearly three million Americans suffer from rheumatoid arthritis, and most are helped by the use of steroid injections, aspirin, and nonsteroidal anti-inflammatories like Advil and Aleve. The relatively new nonsteroidal anti-inflammatory cyclooxygenate inhibitor or Cox-2 inhibitor, such as Celebrex, has been found to relieve pain without many of the typical side effects of other nonsteroidals. This means it can be used in higher doses than other nonsteroidals, simply providing more pain relief for arthritis patients.

Exercise and physical therapy are vital to all arthritis patients, because in addition to maintaining healthy bones, they strengthen the muscles around the joints, enabling them to take on more of the burden of body functioning. Diet is also an important element in the arthritis maintenance program. If your regular health-care provider is not reaching ample pain relief for your arthritis, try glucosamine chondroitin and consult a pain-management specialist.

BACK PAIN

Lower back pain is one of the most common ailments among adults, from all walks of life. Lower back pain can result from a wide variety of causes and, if it becomes chronic, it is usually due to a combination of factors that alter with the passage of time. This means that the proper treatment will vary, depending on the current state of your syndrome.

Lower back pain is divided into two categories. Pain that remains in the general area of the lower back is typically muscle pain (also known as myofascial pain). Back pain accompanied by the extra component of shooting pain into the extremities, such as the legs, is a nerve pain. This section addresses the first kind of lower back problem, myofascial pain. The shooting nerve pain is discussed below, under Back Pain with Radiation.

Myofascial Back Pain

Myofascial lower back pain, the syndrome that remains in the lower back area, is a spasm of the muscles in the lower back. There are about fifteen muscles in the lower back, reaching between the pelvis and the spine. If you overtax one of them, or make it do something it doesn't have the natural ability to do, it will contract into a defensive position and won't release. Although you might be able to tell which side is having a spasm, it's hard to tell exactly which muscle it is. This simple spasm can cause some of the most debilitating pain imaginable, a wrenching lock that can affect every movement, since the lower back is the focal point of most body motion.

Over time, this grip even recruits additional muscles nearby to spasm as well, even the muscles all the way up the spine into the upper back. Substance P and lactic acid released by a spasmodic muscle will also encourage these nearby muscles to spasm by irritating them. In addition to the muscle spasm, the body tries to compensate by adjusting its posture, tilting the hips or rolling to one side as you walk. This aggravates the muscles on the healthy side— and they may start to spasm as well. Soon it is more and more difficult for this patient to sit, stand, or sleep comfortably. It becomes a vicious cycle that only grows more painful unless it is treated.

Because the back is the focal point for all body motion, any activity causes extreme pain. Even resting in bed does not allow the muscles to relax. Muscles only relax completely when the body is in REM (rapid eye movement) sleep, the cycle that is reached after three to four hours of uninterrupted sleep. If a patient awakens every two hours because of the pain, she is never getting to REM sleep. She sleeps with twelve pillows, in a chair, anyplace she can find a comfortable spot, and still doesn't reach that REM sleep stage, which is so important to the healing of myofascial pain.

Between its tendencies to spread and to create an inability to get proper rest, myofascial pain can increase with time and turn the original lower back spasm into a monster of a pain syndrome. This is one of the documented ways a patient develops fibromyalgia.

The typical person most likely to experience a spasm in the lower back is someone who was once in good shape but who has fallen out of condition. As a person ages, he loses muscle mass—his muscles thin out and get weaker—but he might still be doing the same level of activity from his younger days. This might be the "weekend warrior," someone who is inactive most of the week and then devotes a single day to mowing the lawn, working out at the club, and then riding in a bike race. There is no single activity in particular that causes a lower back muscle to spasm, simply too much exercise in an area with too little muscle bulk to handle the task.

The stability of the lower back also relies on the relationship between the lower back muscles and the abdominal muscles. Weak abs or being overweight with underdeveloped abdominal muscles will cause an imbalance that taxes the lower back muscles. They are forced to operate in a way they weren't designed to handle. Someone carrying too much weight where he or she normally doesn't, such as a pregnant woman or a man carrying a heavy briefcase, will lean more in one direction to balance weight distribution, straining back muscles. This will create an imbalance in the lower back, which can cause muscles to spasm during a normally easy task, such as lifting a suitcase into a car or picking up a small child. Once a spasm occurs, it can resolve itself spontaneously, or linger for a few days before going away, or get worse until it is a chronic back pain. The longer the back pain stays, the more difficult it is to heal. Muscle memory enters the scenario, holding the patient in a locked spasm posture. This initial spasmodic muscle can occur in several areas: the upper back, the back of the neck, the shoulders, and the legs. The most common location is in the lower back.

Treatments for this pain syndrome are focused on

relieving the spasm and reducing the inflamed muscle. This is achieved by a combination including muscle relaxants and nonsteroidal anti-inflammatory medication. If the spasm is localized to a single area, then a trigger-point steroid injection can bring quick relief and stop it from becoming a larger syndrome. Hot and cold packs are helpful, as is the TENS treatment we described on page 112. The severity and time lapse of the pain help determine what kind of doctor should treat it. For an acute spasm, a primary-care physician can prescribe the right combination of medications, trigger-point injections, or acupuncture. If the pain state becomes chronic, then more aggressive therapy will be required, including plenty of physical therapy to retrain healthy muscle memory. The chronic syndrome requires a pain-management specialist and a physical therapy center for treatment.

Back Pain with Radiation

The second category of lower back pain is the deep, sharp-shooting pain radiating from the back and down one or both legs. Also known as radicular pain, this is caused by injury to nerves rather than muscles. A herniated disc causes the most common nerve pain—and it's becoming more common with gym-going baby boomers.

The bones of the spine keep us balanced upright on two feet, and they connect through the sacrum and sacroiliac joints to the pelvis. The weight of the upper body travels the length of the spine until it reaches this point, where the weight is transferred to the legs. Discs are the soft-cored leathery cushions between vertebrae, the bones of the spine. They are used every time you walk, sit, bend, twist, for almost every body movement. A herniated (from the Latin for *ruptured*) disc occurs when the gelatinous disc between two vertebrae pops out of its exterior membrane, like the insides of a well-roasted marshmallow. Carrying a heavy weight or even a subtle twist can make the disc burst its invisible seams. Most herniated discs occur in the lumbar, or lower spine area, and don't cause any pain at all. In fact, many people right now—roughly 30 percent of all adults—are walking around with no idea that they have one or more herniated discs. But when a herniated disc hits a nerve root, you most certainly feel pain. A *lot* of pain—like having an exposed nerve when you lose a filling in your tooth. This back pain, called lumbar radiculopathy, is much greater because the nerves in the lower back are the largest in the body. It is sometimes caused by other pain syndromes such as spinal stenosis.

In addition, herniated discs can cause pain elsewhere in the body, in the places served by the nerve root that is irritated. A shooting nerve pain in the arm, for example, might be caused by a herniated disc in the upper vertebrae of the neck. Known as cervical radiculopathy, this is often what people refer to when they have "whiplash." The pain of herniated discs also affects nerves that go to the muscles of the spine. Therefore, all the conditions of myofascial back pain, described above, frequently accompany radicular pain.

The nerve roots for the legs pass through the spinal column, as do all the body's nerve roots. When a nerve root is damaged in the lower spinal area, it might be one of the leg's nerve roots that feed into the sciatic nerve. This pain is called sciatica. Even though the injury might be in the spinal area, the leg's nerve root is telling the brain that the leg hurts. This is perceived by the patient as deep shooting pain all the way down the back of her leg to her toes, in addition to the pain in the lower back.

A different cause of nerve pain in the lower back is facet joint inflammation. The bones of the spine rest on facets called zygapophyseal joints that allow a person to bend and twist. An aging person might get arthritis here, inflaming the joints and causing them to hit a nerve that also goes down the leg. A twist injury can also inflame the sacroiliac joint in an elderly person, creating a lot of pain. This kind of pain usually does not extend below the knees and is frequently visible in an MRI, where you can observe the changes in the facet joint.

The third area that can cause radicular pain is inflammation of the piriformis muscle. The piriformis muscle is in the sciatic "notch," a large muscle that almost resembles a pair of trousers. This is usually diagnosed by a process of elimination, when the radicular pain is not emanating from a herniated disc or facet joint.

As people reach their sixties and seventies, it is common for their spinal canals to become narrower. This is known as spinal stenosis, and it aggravates the lower back nerves, crowding them in the spinal canal. This slow onset of nerve pain aches through the lower back and legs, eventually inhibiting the patient's ability to walk.

As you can see, there are a number of spots along the spinal nerves that, when inflamed, can radiate pain down the legs. Lumbar radiculopathy and cervical radiculopathy can be treated successfully—without surgery—in about 75 percent of all patients. Treatment of radiating back pain depends on the individual case. If it is a herniated disc, then an epidural steroid injection is the primary choice for most effective healing. However, some patients prefer a more conservative treatment than injection. Many prefer oral medications for disc pain, such as tricyclic antidepressants, even though they will take longer and they are not as potent in the body by the time they reach the pain. If it is a facet joint pain, then an injection into the joint can reduce inflammation and, therefore, reduce the pain. Pain in the sacroiliac joints or in the piriformis muscle responds well to an injection of a steroid and local anesthetic. After the pain is reduced, the patient must begin a physical therapy program to strengthen the affected muscles and prevent the pain from returning.

Patients with radiating back pain must be treated quickly by a physician who is experienced enough to diagnose it. This kind of back pain almost always requires an MRI to assist in the diagnosis. Some patients may discover that the disc is compromising an important nerve, and the hernia must be surgically removed as quickly as possible, before permanent damage sets in. Surgery is necessary for less than 20 percent of my patients who have herniated discs. But it is important to remember that the timeliness of correct treatment is required to prevent permanent nerve damage. And back pain with radiation is never completely cured unless injections and overlapping medications are used as part of the complete Painbuster four-step program.

BROKEN BONE

See Traumatic Injury.

BURSITIS

A bursa is a fluid-filled sac that helps your tendons and bones work together. There are dozens of them throughout your body, although the most common in pain cases are in the shoulder or the knee. Once in a while, a bursa might become swollen from some sort of fluid accumulation, caused by anything from an infection to an injury that makes pus form there. The bursa becomes distended and very painful. Our primary goal is to reduce the inflammation, which will then reduce the pain. The swelling can often be reduced merely by pressing heat packs directly over the area, supported by taking a nonsteroidal anti-inflammatory. In fact, almost all bursitis cases can be resolved with this rather conservative method. Otherwise, using a hypodermic needle simply to draw out the fluid can achieve the same effect. But unless you uncover what is causing the fluid, it will just start accumulating again.

CANCER

Cancer pain is one of the most undertreated in the field of medicine. Not only does the patient have a disease that brings her to the brink of mortality, but she has progressively worsening pain that can limit her functioning, even if she beats the disease. Studies show that most patients diagnosed with cancer expect to experience intractable pain during the course of the disease. And they do. Most of us have known someone who has experienced this excruciating pain. Part of the despair associated with the diagnosis of cancer is the fear of pain, a fear that is based on a grim reality. Cancer causes pain.

There is no other symptom of a disease treated with quite the same disregard as pain is. If someone expects to experience high blood pressure during the course of an illness, the patient does not usually accept it as unavoidable. He knows it can be controlled with medication, because such medications exist. Patients don't think twice about taking medication to control high blood pressure. Yet cancer patients seem to expect that they will have to endure agonizing pain without sufficient medications. This philosophy belongs in the annals of the Dark Ages, along with bleeding purges and blister therapy. I cannot explain why health-care providers perpetuate the gloomy prognosis of cancer pain in this era, when it can be completely and safely prevented. Perhaps it is simply because they are not yet comfortable treating pain. Perhaps it is because pain is so difficult to measure, being as subjective as it is. What causes pain in one person may have no effect in another. Perhaps it is because there is still a stigma attached to certain prescription pain medications, a stigma both in the mind of the health-care provider and in the mind of the patient. These are only my best guesses. But I know cancer patients feel intense pain, and it is traditionally undertreated.

In cancer treatment, all the types of pain usually enter

the equation. If a tumor grows against bone, it will produce a different kind of pain than if it grows against a nerve. When a tumor starts obstructing organs, it will create a variety of pain types. Obstruction of the ureter, the tube that carries urine from the kidneys to the bladder, causes what we call "flank" pain. Flank pain is eliminated by treating the underlying cause of pain—in this case, the obstruction. If a tumor is obstructing a blood vessel, then the area served by that blood vessel will begin to lose oxygen and nutrients. This is called ischemic pain, which might manifest itself in a part of the body far from where the actual obstruction is, sending pain signals to the brain because it is languishing without oxygen. Just about the only place a growing tumor doesn't hurt is in the brain. The brain has no pain receptors.

Additional pain might also derive from surgery or procedures used to combat the cancer, from the treatment's side effects (alongside nausea or constipation), or, not least of all, from the psychological effects of having the disease in the first place. In order to treat the cancer patient properly, all of these elements need to be explored. This can be a great challenge, because the nature of the pain frequently changes during the course of this disease and its treatment.

The second most significant cause of cancer pain comes from the treatments used to stop the disease. The same is true for HIV pain. Medications to fight cancer and HIV are very potent and toxic, with long lists of side effects. They are usually targeted to specific areas, but they frequently affect other systems in the body. Small nerve fibers of the central nervous system are particularly susceptible to pain from cancer treatments. Radiation therapy causes pain because it destroys tissue. Some of it is cancerous, but some of the surrounding tissue it destroys is healthy, and that hurts. This burning sensation from the injury of small nerve fibers might be restricted to one part of the body, but it can extend much farther than the tumor itself.

Over time, as the patient's health and activity level change, the types of pain change, too. They must be assessed frequently, and the treatment altered accordingly. The patient is already on a complex medication regimen to control the cancer. Adding more medications for pain can exacerbate the side effects of all of them. For example, most pain medications are somewhat sedating. If a patient is already drowsy from cancer drugs, then certain pain medications will make this problem worse. Sometimes, a cancer patient whose pain is being successfully managed might need an emergency surgery, which will throw the whole pain-management regimen for a loop, and which will require extra methods to regain control. There is a fine dynamic in the treatment of cancer pain, in its many variations and stages, requiring constant communication between doctors to stay one step ahead of the pain.

In addition to pain caused by medical side effects, the dismantling of a tumor in itself will cause pain. When medications cause tumorous masses to break down, these masses are dispersed into the body. When the products of this breakdown flow through the bloodstream, it hurts. Depending on the size of the tumor, and the speed at which it breaks down in the body, the resulting pain can vary. Certain combinations of cancer medications can also cause a general neuropathy, or nerve pain, throughout the entire body.

One of the greatest influences on cancer pain is psychological treatment. Stress, the anticipation of cancer pain, and a sense of helplessness in fighting this disease make it very difficult for a patient to maintain a positive outlook, to say the least. Of course, cancer pain management is a highly personalized treatment. Many patients are embarrassed to admit they even have pain, because they don't want to discourage their oncologists who are working so hard to control the cancer. But a patient and doctor should know that efforts can be made to control pain, that there are resources available for that specific pain treatment from health-care providers whom they can trust. Sufficient pain control might even help the patient to begin cancer treatment with more confidence, strength, and hope.

The medical treatment for cancer pain focuses on breaking down the causes of the pain. First, I obtain a comprehensive pain history from the patient and determine what types of pain are involved. If it is small nerve irritation from radiation, then a neuropathic pain medication like Neurontin might be appropriate. If it is pressure on a nerve, such as a metastatic lesion pressing on a rib, then we might treat this cancer pain as we do other intercostal pain. If the pain involves a multitude of symptoms and is widespread, then we might opt for a chronic narcotic therapy, such as the intrathecal infusion device, described on page 77. As with most pain syndromes, we have found that the most effective treatment for cancer pain is a combination of medications.

Your oncologist is the first person to consult about pain-management therapies. These doctors are familiar with many pain treatments and can usually initiate the treatment successfully. If the pain worsens or becomes too difficult to control, request an evaluation from a pain-management specialist. This allows the oncologist to focus on treating the cancer, while the pain specialist focuses on the pain. In most cases, the pain-management specialist need only be consulted intermittently while the oncologist maintains the patient's cancer regimen. If the pain worsens, or the cancer is terminal, the pain-management specialist can become part of the team that provides palliative care, for pain control during the end of life, which is described in chapter 9.

CARPAL TUNNEL SYNDROME

There are no muscles in the wrist, but there are five long tendons that travel through the wrist as they connect the finger muscles to the arm muscles. The bones of the wrist are called the carpus, and these long tendons run right through what is called the carpal tunnel. When these tendons become chronically inflamed, the wrist is very painful. This disease occurs most frequently in women, and it has been known to be affected by hormone levels and sports injuries, but most cases of this syndrome can be directly attributed to repetitive motion. Those with jobs that require constant tasks using their hands—such as hairstylists, assembly-line workers, and anyone who uses a computer keyboard—are the most common victims of this ailment.

The inflammation of the tendons can be controlled by a trigger-point injection of a steroid compound. I have also seen acupuncture work wonders on this syndrome. A brace on the wrist might help keep inflammation reduced. If none of these is helpful, I would turn to surgery as a last resort, to widen the tunnel so that inflamed tendons no longer cause pain. Interestingly, I have frequently observed this syndrome fade away in a few weeks on its own, without any treatment at all.

CAUSALGIA

See Complex Regional Pain Syndrome, Type I.

CENTRAL PAIN SYNDROME

This disease often strikes between three and nine months after a stroke or an injury to the circulation system. Central pain syndrome feels like arthritis pain—aches in the joints—except that they are limited to the side affected by the stroke. Since the pain appears in parts of the body that have already lost some function, the patient is sometimes confused by the cause of this pain, and it inhibits most occupational therapy or physical therapy in the affected areas.

We call this one a diagnosis of exclusion, meaning that all other diseases must be ruled out—primarily complex regional pain syndrome and arthritis—before we diagnose central pain syndrome. The only cure to this syndrome is to treat the symptoms, which are a combination of nerve pain and bony pain. I have found that, unlike complex regional pain syndrome, this disease does not respond to injection therapy. Medications that work the best are a combination of nonsteroidal anti-inflammatories, nerve pain agents such as tricyclic antidepressants for the large nerve pain, and narcotics. Once the pain is under control, it is unlikely to return.

The neurologist who treats the stroke patient should be able to treat central pain syndrome, although that doctor may want the patient to consult a pain-management specialist. Naturally, the neurologist would also work with the patient for preventative maintenance against future strokes, and physical therapy to regain normal functions.

COMPLEX REGIONAL PAIN SYNDROME (CRPS), TYPE I

This disease of the central nervous system was known as causalgia for many years. This is the pain from direct nerve damage, such as an injury or trauma. This direct injury is how Type I is distinguished from CRPS Type II, which is caused by something other than direct nerve injury. The first line of treatment for Type I is to reverse the damage that is causing the problem: to repair the nerve, either through surgery or traction. Then one can address the pain caused by the sympathetic nerves, which is addressed under the syndrome described immediately below.

COMPLEX REGIONAL PAIN SYNDROME (CRPS), TYPE II

This disease has had many names, most recently sympathetically mediated pain and reflex sympathetic dystrophy (RSD), and it is sometimes mistaken for causalgia (Type I). The difference is that CRPS Type II occurs even when there has been no nerve injury. This was the syndrome first described by Silas Weir Mitchell during the Civil War. He found that, even in cases where there was no direct nerve damage, some patients suffered intolerable, intense pain in extremities that were not even wounded. Weir Mitchell developed ways to distinguish this very real pain from other war trauma effects, such as anxiety and deluded memory. During all the time since his discovery, the actual cause of this pain syndrome has eluded researchers.

Most health-care providers are not very familiar with this disease, which means it can take a long time for the CRPS sufferer to get a proper diagnosis. Therefore, it is not unusual to obtain correct treatment long after the initial phases of this disease, which, not surprisingly, slows the cure. Early treatment is the key to success.

The classic symptoms of this disease are unique, so CRPS is usually not confused with any other syndrome. After a minor injury or surgery, in most cases the original pain recedes. But within a couple of weeks, a new, more intense pain takes its place. This is called Stage 1, typified by a swelling in an arm or leg, at first intensely red, then perhaps intermittent changing to white or a bluish color. The swelling is hot; the patient sweats profusely. The natural pain transmitters are simply in overdrive.

In Stage 2, a light touch over the affected area causes a severe burning pain. We call this kind of pain allodynia, and it is unusual because it is a reaction to a pain stimulus that doesn't exist. A CRPS patient finds even a bedsheet too painful to cover the area, and clothing can feel unbearable. A breeze or slight chill causes further discomfort. Because of the pain and swelling, the patient loses function of this extremity, trying to protect it from touching anything. What has happened is that, in addition to the transmitters, now the receptors have started to increase in number. When you have developed too many receptors, they do not go away. These symptoms continue indefinitely and may enter a new phase, which we call brawny edema, where the swelling becomes cold and hard to the touch. Over the course of six months or as long as two years, hair stops growing over the affected area, the joints move less and less, and muscle tone begins to disappear due to inactivity.

If allowed to progress to Stage 3, CRPS is a devastating condition. All the changes are permanent. The joints are fused in a locked position, the muscle virtually disappears. The tiniest movement can trigger acute pains. Some patients in Stage 3 even choose to have the afflicted extremities amputated. Identifying CRPS early is imperative to preventing Stage 3.

Although the cause for this disease is not known, there appears to be a link between the sympathetic nervous system and the sensory nerve system. The sensory nerve feels a pain message, bringing stress to the body, causing the sympathetic nerves to respond and transmit more pain messages to the sensory nerves, and so on. The nerves are constantly telling the brain they feel pain, causing stress on the body and a vicious pain cycle. The best treatment is aimed at stopping the endless loop of pain messages.

The only way to test for CRPS is to perform a sympathetic nerve block. In other words, block the sympathetic nerves in the affected area for a short period of time. If the symptoms go away, then this patient has CRPS. If the pain remains, even after the blockade of a sympathetic nerve, then it is not CRPS. Other syndromes must then be pursued, such as central pain syndrome, nerve damage, or surgical scarring. It is important to perform this sympathetic nerve block before any other treatment, so that you know what you're treating.

The cure for CRPS is physical therapy, combined with physical therapy and more physical therapy. This area must be returned to normal function as quickly as possible. This is the only treatment that consistently brings success. But how can the patient do physical therapy if the area hurts so much? By continuing to block the sympathetic nerves, as in the original diagnostic test. This is why a pain-management specialist is the ideal doctor to supervise treatment. Since physical therapy is the only antidote to this condition, all we do is use medications and injections to get the pain under control and get the patient into physical therapy.

There are several ways to block sympathetic nerves. The least invasive method is a series of sympathetic nerve block injections. These injections of local anesthetic into the body provide complete relief for a period of time, and the pain relief lasts longer after each treatment. For the upper extremities, the injection goes into the neck, where the sympathetic nerves of the upper extremities merge together. For the lower extremities, the injection needs to go just outside the spinal column, on the front side of the vertebrae, so the needle goes through the front of the body. Then the patient performs aggressive physical therapy while the pain reliever is in effect, which should be for several days.

The next least invasive treatment is to insert an epidural catheter for a couple of days, offering a continuous infusion of local anesthetic. This blocks the sympathetic nerves long enough for them to "reset" themselves to a normal, pain-free status. Unfortunately, this usually requires the patient to stay in a hospital during that time, and somehow still maintain a physical therapy regimen. An alternative to this method is the bretylium bier blockade, a delivery method that allows for outpatient treatment. Bretylium is a synthetic replacement for the neurotransmitter, norepinephrine, essentially cutting off the pain-message loop until the body has enough time to replenish its own norepinephrine. This blockade involves the inflation of a tourniquet on the affected limb, and infusing the vessels with the bretylium (or with a similar medication called guanethidine). The nerves are all around these vessels, and the medication leeches through into the afflicted nerves. After less than sixty minutes of such infusion, the sympathetic nervous system will stop transmitting pain messages, and the relief might last several weeks. This allows for a great deal of physical therapy in the meantime.

Should none of these treatments provide long-term relief, I recommend moving on to spinal cord stimulation, which will stop the pain in about 75 percent of CRPS patients. We would use this treatment with every CRPS patient, but it is a fairly invasive procedure, as explained in chapter 8. Some doctors advocate the use of ablations of sympathetic nerves for CRPS—the surgical removal of the painful section of a sympathetic nerve—but I do not think ablations are the best approach in these cases. Ablations cause permanent change in the sympathetic system, and I see no reason to go to this extreme when other, less invasive, procedures might also work.

However the patient reaches pain relief, it will not last forever. Most of the treatments, with the exception of spinal cord stimulation, will only block the pain transmitters for a short time. Physical therapy is what has the lasting effect. Psychological counseling can also be important for the cure of CRPS. It helps reduce stress during treatment and physical therapy and lessen the general despair caused by such a frustrating pain condition. Because early diagnosis and treatment are key to the cure of CRPS, you need a physician who is familiar with this disease, and who can perform the necessary procedures. A neurologist working with a physical therapist can manage this syndrome, but a pain-management specialist is recommended to implement the nerve block injections.

DIABETIC POLYNEUROPATHY

This pain state has consistent symptoms, in what a doctor would call a classic presentation. With the onset of diabetes, many patients develop a burning pain in the feet and hands, known as the stocking-glove distribution of pain. This searing pain is constant and worsens with time. It is uncertain exactly what causes this pain, but we believe it is due to decreased blood flow to the small nerve endings in the affected area. This small nerve pain can occur even when the diabetes is being successfully controlled.

There are very few medications to which this syndrome responds. But I have found that the antiarrhythmic heart medication Mexitil (mexilitine) is very effective, particularly when it is combined with a nonsteroidal anti-inflammatory like Motrin. Of course, the patient should be evaluated to assure that an antiarrhythmic will not adversely affect her cardiac status. In nearly every instance I have observed, Mexitil has completely relieved the pain of diabetic neuropathy when other medications have failed. The physician who treats your diabetes should be comfortable using this medication to treat the pain.

FIBROMYALGIA

This is a very challenging pain syndrome, with multiple symptoms that change over time. There are no specific tests to diagnose fibromyalgia, which is also known as fibrositis, chronic rheumatism, myofascial pain syndrome, pressure point syndrome, or psychogenic arthritis. The cause is rarely found, although we have identified a constellation of other diseases that are associated with it, such as arthritis, multiple sclerosis, chronic fatigue syndrome, and large nerve pains such as tennis elbow. The most common symptoms of fibromyalgia (pain of the fibers) are deep muscle aches, morning stiffness, constant fatigue even with adequate sleep, headaches, pain in joints all over the body, and mild bouts of anxiety or depression. Sometimes, a patient suffering from fibromyalgia will also have abdominal pain, frequent urination, swelling or tingling in the hands and feet, and restless sleep. It is estimated that ten million Americans suffer from this pain syndrome. The average fibromyalgia patient is forty-nine years old, and 90 percent of these patients are women.

This pain syndrome often seems to begin during another illness, which we believe contributes to the cause—something like a minor flu, a small injury that doesn't heal, or a stressful emotional trauma. Symptoms get worse, and the patient starts reducing her normal activities. As the symptoms worsen, the patient might isolate herself even more.

The diagnosis of fibromyalgia is based on the presence and location of pain. The standard diagnosis is pain throughout at least half the body; pain in at least eleven out of eighteen specific trigger points; and no other diseases present that would cause this pain. Since pain is the primary symptom of fibromyalgia, successful treatment is focused on reducing the pain, which, in most cases of this disease, is a combination of muscle spasm with bony pain in the joints. It is not uncommon for initial treatments to lose their effectiveness as time passes, so we frequently rotate the medications for a fibromyalgia patient, as frequently as every four weeks. This requires careful record keeping to determine which medications, at which dose, are effective, and which ones do not work.

Returning the patient to normal functioning is essential

to the cure, which is why I treat the symptoms in any way I can to make this happen. In addition to reducing the pain, I also study the patient's sleep cycles to ensure she's getting proper rest. In almost every case, I also recommend stress reduction therapy, perhaps in a group session. Even patients who normally have little stress accumulate more stress when they suffer from fibromyalgia.

Besides rotating the medications and stress therapy, I'll complement the treatment with biofeedback and physical therapy. This is one pain syndrome, however, where it can be harmful to do too much physical activity. Many of these patients were very active before they got fibromyalgia and, therefore, many try to overcompensate after their pain has been reduced. But they are probably no longer in good muscle condition at this point, and too much exercise can lead quickly to an injury and regression to another pain syndrome. I prescribe for these patients some very deliberate and slowly progressive exercises that are designed to increase their strength and flexibility.

Exercises in water are excellent for initial phases of therapy, because this limits the stress on joints and decreases the risk of injury. Walking in chest-high water that is at least eighty-two degrees is ideal. Seek out an aquatic physical therapist or an aquatic instructor who has been certified by the Arthritis Foundation.

More than that, patients who suffer from fibromyalgia need to work with a physician who understands this disease. Other than a pain-management specialist, the specialist who most closely understands fibromyalgia is a rheumatologist.

GOUT

There are many causes of gout, but the pain is always the same. Gout is simply the deposit of a substance into any joint, such as extra uric acid due to a kidney ailment. The substance is very irritating to the joint, causing it to swell and hurt. The pain feels like acute arthritis in the joint, very painful and warm to the touch. The difference is this: Gout pain can start very abruptly, in less than a day. The first thing to do is to remove the irritating substance and its cause, and then treat the pain. By taking a sample of the irritation with a hypodermic needle, and analyzing a small amount of joint fluid, the causative agent can be identified. Then the patient can get the proper medication to stop the overproduction of this substance, and the gout pain usually disappears. Since gout is simple inflammation, it helps to take nonsteroidal anti-inflammatories to ease the pain while the gout is being treated.

HEADACHE

Headaches, although painful, are not usually part of a pain-management specialist's practice. The remedies involve treating the ailment—tension or expansion of the blood vessels in the brain. Minor tension headaches usually disappear on their own, but you could take aspirin or Motrin to soothe the inflamed blood vessels more quickly.

The drugs used for chronic headache, such as migraine, are not the same as those used for pain elsewhere in the body. Treatment and diagnosis for migraine are best performed by a neurologist or headache specialist.

HERPES ZOSTER AND POSTHERPETIC NEURALGIA

These are two different pain syndromes, but they come from the same source. Herpes zoster (better known as shingles) is chicken pox in adults, a derivation of the herpes simplex virus. This virus grows in nerve roots that cover discrete areas of the body, usually on just one side. Almost all patients will have a painful rash over this area of the body, and a doctor can take a sample from this rash to test for the virus. Very few patients do not have a rash with this pain syndrome, but it has been known to happen. The patient has sharp, shooting pains near the rash, from the inflamed nerve roots in the area. We treat this viral infection with medications, usually nonsteroidal anti-inflammatories as well as nerve pain agents, such as tricyclic antidepressants, and the pain goes away. The pain of herpes zoster is rather short-lived, however, and a neuropathic pain agent such as a tricyclic antidepressant can take many days to take effect. If the shingles patient is in a lot of pain and we catch it soon enough, we can speed her pain relief with an epidural injection of steroids around the nerves that serve the rashy area. This soothes the nerve roots inflamed by the infection, bringing immediate pain relief. As with all herpes viruses, the disease treatment is antiviral drugs such as Zovirax and narcotics.

Sometimes we use epidural injections to stop herpes

zoster from progressing into postherpetic neuralgia, which occurs in roughly 50 percent of shingles patients over the age of sixty. This is why herpes zoster must be treated quickly. Postherpetic neuralgia most frequently occurs in elderly patients, or in patients whose immune system has been compromised by another disease. With postherpetic neuralgia, the herpes zoster symptoms go away and are replaced by a new pain, which feels different than the shingles pain. This is a more intense pain in the original area where the rash was, although the rash will be gone by this point. This pain is from the persistent inflammation of the nerve roots in the original herpes area, and it can linger for years.

The foundation of treatment for postherpetic neuralgia is nonsteroidal anti-inflammatories, plus neuropathic pain drugs such as tricyclic antidepressants to calm the inflamed nerves. Epidural steroid injections are very effective in relieving this pain. Nerve block injections are not an option, because this infection lives in the spinal cord, out of reach for injections. Sometimes a topical agent such as Zostrix cream can relieve pain, but it does not provide consistent relief.

These patients usually cannot be cured of the disease; only a few cases show improvement. The best treatment is to reduce the pain, which can be done very effectively by an internist, an infectious disease specialist, or a dermatologist. Since nerve pain medications and epidural injections are standard treatments, you should consult a doctor who is very familiar with these pain relief procedures.

HIV

Like cancer pain, the human immunodeficiency virus (HIV) is a disease whose pain is very undertreated. Actually, the pain symptoms of cancer are very similar to those of HIV and the AIDS (acquired immune deficiency syndrome) virus. A secondary infection, or a tumor growth like Kaposi's sarcoma, will cause intense pain. A tumor growth in, say, the abdomen, might continue growing until it is pressing against the organs there, prohibiting their function as well as causing pain. It is not always clear which will happen first—whether pain will arrive before or after a tumor impedes an organ's functions. If the tumor is in the capsule holding the liver, then it's likely to cause pain before a liver malfunction. A tumor in the abdomen, however, may have plenty of room to grow before it begins to be painful.

We frequently see HIV patients with widespread nerve pain caused by viruses other than the HIV. The pain syndrome of herpes zoster, for example, is usually found in older HIV patients, and postherpetic neuralgia can appear in anyone whose immune system is compromised. Many times, the cause of HIV nerve pain cannot be identified, but the pain is there.

As with cancer pain, HIV pain can result from the medical treatments for the disease. Newer treatments for HIV, such as specific antiviral agents, are known to cause severe arthritis-type symptoms. It is suspected that these drugs also irritate the lining of the lungs, an inflammation that makes every breath painful. In addition, other side effects from HIV treatments may make a patient uncomfortable; nausea, diarrhea, constipation, and sedation can aggravate a patient's condition. Pain management can be used to alleviate them all.

We use both traditional medications for nerve pain for many HIV patients and, sometimes, acupuncture to maximize pain relief with minimal side effects. We also rely on psychological treatments to control HIV pain. I have observed great pain relief for HIV patients when psychological counseling is an integral part of the treatment program. Sufferers know their symptoms "must" include pain, and the counseling helps them adjust their outlook. As with cancer patients, the pain treatments for those with HIV must be constantly reevaluated to follow the patient's particular symptoms. With all the resources available today, no HIV patient should settle for pain in any stage of the disease.

In most cases, the pain treatment of HIV-related pain can be provided by the patient's primary-care provider. If the pain becomes difficult to control, then it would help to consult a pain specialist for suggestions. Because the drug regimens are complicated, good communication among the physicians is essential. Most of the time, a stable pain regimen can be achieved that can then be maintained by the primary-care provider.

INTERCOSTAL NEURITIS

Most people have never heard of this pain syndrome, but when they hear the symptoms, they recognize intercostal neuritis. It is a sharp nerve pain that shoots along the rib cage, from your back around to the front of your chest.

Under each rib is a sort of coaxial cable of nerve, vein, and artery, running along the lower edge of each rib, from the spine all the way around the front, to the center of your chest. The intercostal nerve in this cable can be irritated by a number of causes: a broken rib, surgical removal of a rib, or a mass pressing into the nerve. Touching this area can reproduce the shooting pain, but it will usually cause plenty of pain without touching it at all. Even though this pain is very uncomfortable, the more important concern is that it can disrupt normal breathing—every breath causes a deep pain.

A fractured rib will heal within several days, but sometimes when the nerve has been disrupted or injured, this acute bony-nerve pain combination can become chronic. If the pain is mild, it is best treated with a nonsteroidal anti-inflammatory, combined with a tricyclic antidepressant. If pain persists, then I would recommend a nerve block injection of a local anesthetic, one that will numb the nerve long enough to heal itself. If the local anesthetic is helpful, but the nerve continues to be painful without the injection long after the injury, then the patient and doctor might consider an advanced ablation, such as cryoablation. Cryoablation freezes the injured nerve, essentially destroying it, but allows regrowth of the nerve without the pain. Nerves are so slow to regenerate that, by the time they return to normal, the original cause of the pain is long gone. For hospitalized patients with multiple broken ribs, an epidural catheter with a local anesthetic will numb the nerves over a large area, and a small amount of narcotics will reduce pain and enable the patient to take normal breaths.

These treatments are usually performed by a pain-management specialist or an anesthesiologist. Your primary-care physician should seek out one of these specialists to help resolve intercostal neuritis.

ISCHEMIA OR ISCHEMIC PAIN

See Vascular Pain.

KIDNEY STONES

See Traumatic Injury.

OBSTETRIC PAIN

There are a number of acute pains that can occur during the course of a woman's pregnancy—for example, lower back muscle pain caused by her added girth, sciatica, or perhaps a broken toe. But traditional pain relief during a pregnancy is very conservative, because anything that enters the woman's system will also affect her unborn baby. The pregnant woman's body usually compensates for this because it's already increasing its production of natural endorphins, in anticipation of childbirth. Endorphins relieve a woman's childbirth pain naturally, if not always entirely. If only other patients could produce as much pain relief as a pregnant woman!

Acute back pain is a common occurrence in pregnant women. As her baby develops, the mother's center of gravity changes. A woman weighs more during pregnancy than she will probably weigh in her lifetime, which, in itself, is an added stress to her body. On top of that, most of it is concentrated on her abdomen. This added girth is carried in front of her normal pivot points, the pelvis and lower back. The posture of a pregnant woman tends to lean back slightly, to distribute her weight more evenly. To counteract the extra weight in the abdomen, her lower back muscles pick up some of the added effort. If a woman gains weight over a longer period of time, her back muscles would have a chance to strengthen and handle this new task. But in only a few weeks, the back is called upon to compensate rather quickly. Also, as noted in the section on back pain, the abdominal muscles are important for stabilizing the lower back. When the abs are stretched out during pregnancy, they are much less helpful in supporting the lower back. A woman with any risk of normal back pain will surely feel it during pregnancy.

Sometimes, a pregnant mother in a painful situation is better off taking additional pain medication. For example, if the patient develops a kidney stone, the stress from her uncontrolled pain will be worse for the unborn baby than the effects of certain pain relievers. We always select pain relievers that have an established track record in pregnant women, and we minimize the number of different medications we usually use in pain treatment.

Most pain medications are harmful to developing infants. The risks simply outweigh the benefits. Benzodiazapines such as Valium and Xanax have been known to cause birth defects and are never used in pregnant women. Nonsteroidal anti-inflammatories can change the blood flow to an embryo, so they are also rarely used. However, Tylenol has proved to be relatively safe for pregnant patients. The more developed the fetus, the better able it is to cope with a mother's pain medication. Another option for a pregnant woman in chronic acute pain is narcotics therapy. This medication will cross into the baby's system as well, but it can be carefully tapered off after delivery, with no lasting side effects at all. Naturally, this must be done under close medical supervision, but narcotics are a safe alternative for both mother and baby.

There are two kinds of pain involved in childbirth itself. The first is the pain of labor, which is the contraction of the uterus, a large muscle spasm not unlike a charley horse. A labor contraction, however, occurs repeatedly every few minutes, over the course of several hours. The second type of childbirth pain occurs when the baby passes through the birth canal. Like the contractions, this event is not particularly comfortable. But the good news with obstetric pain is that the patient usually has had five or six months to investigate her pain-management options before she needs them. She is one of the best-educated consumers we meet, because she usually does her homework about anesthetics for when her time comes. I encourage you to explore the choices available at the local facility where you plan to give birth. The options are not the same from one place to another. The facility should be happy to explain to you the various options it can provide.

Throughout history, women have successfully used techniques like breathing exercises and focused concentration to control their labor pain. This is based on the premise that concentrating on something other than the contractions will distract the mother from pain. There are no side effects to this mind-over-matter principle of pain relief, and it helps many women feel better. But there is no guarantee that this method will work for every patient. Most women do not know, in advance, if breathing will provide enough pain relief for them. But because this technique has no side effects, it is a good option to start with. If this method is not successful in controlling the pain of contractions, however, it is best to have another option to fall back on. Acupuncture is the least invasive alternative, but not many hospitals provide acupuncturists in the delivery room, and some patients do not respond to this method of treatment.

Medications have been used for years to decrease the pain of labor and delivery. Ideally, the medication would make the mother comfortable, yet still allow her to fully participate in the process. This can be a challenge since some of our usual pain-relieving medications cause sedation or confusion. After all the time and energy a woman has spent on her pregnancy and the anticipation of her new baby, the last thing you want to do is sedate the mother so much that she doesn't remember the birth itself. In the delivery room, the most commonly used pain relievers are intravenous narcotics, which are the quickest-acting on all types of pain. They must be used judiciously to avoid oversedation. Another common procedure for obstetric pain is a labor epidural. Anesthesiologists call this method "central access medication." Unlike intravenous narcotics, the epidural injection controls the pain precisely in the area where the pain exists, in the nerve roots as they exit from the lower spine. By placing medication near these nerves, even just small amounts, the pain is controlled.

There are two different medications commonly used in an epidural injection: local anesthetics and narcotics. The local anesthetic, such as Xylocaine (lidocaine), decreases the nerve's ability to send pain messages. Thus, the sensation of contraction pain is greatly reduced. The local anesthetic can be administered periodically over the course of labor and delivery, every time the pain returns, or even as a continuous infusion to keep the pain away. The drawback to this pain relief method is that a professional needs to administer it and monitor this medication, and not all hospitals provide this service. Local anesthetics can also cause weakness in the leg and abdominal muscles, which are needed for the delivery process. Used correctly, however, local anesthetics are an excellent pain reliever. They allow the mother to feel contractions, without pain, and retain the strength to push when the time comes.

Narcotics may also be injected into the epidural space, in combination with the local anesthetic. Narcotics such as morphine or fentanyl reduce the pain through a different mechanism. This combination was introduced so that the amount of local anesthetic could be reduced. Both require lower doses than if one was used alone. Narcotics enhance the effects of the local anesthetic while reducing its side effects. Some people call this combination a "walking epidural," because it does not affect the use of one's legs.

The goal of controlling obstetric pain is to reduce the pain of contractions without blocking all sensations or body strength. Whatever methods make you comfortable are the ones you should choose. Investigate the options at your local hospital and determine what will work for you.

PELVIC PAIN

As with abdominal pain, the structure of the pelvis makes it difficult to pinpoint the exact cause of pain. Chronic pelvic pain has similar symptoms as abdominal pain—a pervasive ache—only it might also be exacerbated by menstrual pains or changes in bowel function. A thorough exam by a gynecologist is essential for women with pelvic pain, because it often signals the presence of fibroid tumors in the uterus or a bladder infection.

The treatment is similar to that for abdominal pain, including medication with nerve pain drugs or long-acting narcotics. This syndrome can also be relieved with a nerve block injection in the superior hypogastric plexus, which is the nerve center transversed by all the pelvic nerves. This pain syndrome is often associated with emotional factors, such as relationship problems, so I would also recommend consulting a psychologist to obtain an accurate diagnosis and treatment.

PHANTOM LIMB PAIN

There are three categories of sensation that affect patients who have had an amputation. The first kind is the stump pain, the postsurgical scar pain on the stump. Stump pain lasts longer than other kinds of postoperative pain, because there are a variety of sources, depending on the general condition and the particular procedure. Sometimes the stump pain is caused by a neuroma formation at the surgery site, which is a tip of the nerve that grows into a ball, and it is painful when touched. There might be a bony irritation if the tissue covering the bone is not thick enough, or ischemic pain if there is not enough blood flow to the area. Recognizing the differences among each of these problems enables a doctor to repair the cause of pain, either with a surgical revision of the stump, or a specially modified prosthesis.

The second phenomenon of an amputation is the phantom limb sensation. This is not necessarily pain, but the sensation that the removed body part is still there. The patient senses the extremity is in a normal position, and it feels just as it used to, even though it is gone. Most patients sense this after an amputation. For some people, however, the phantom limb sensation is excruciating pain.

Phantom limb pain is a bizarre condition that sometimes appears within four weeks of an amputation, although it has been known to arrive more than a year later. The patient feels as if the missing extremity is being crushed, twisted, or contorted into an unnatural position. This pain is constant and chronic. In rare cases, this pain will resolve itself and fade away over time. There are no specific treatments that are overwhelmingly successful with phantom limb pain. What works for one patient may have absolutely no effect on another. Therefore, the trial and error of an individualized plan is the best approach. In my experience, irreversible techniques such as nerve ablations and stump revisions do not have any effect on phantom limb pain. I have seen some improvements using reversible techniques, such as epidural infusion and spinal cord stimulation. But the best effects I have seen are with medication management, and I have found the most success using neuropathic agents such as tricyclic antidepressants.

POSTOPERATIVE PAIN

Having surgery is as traumatic to your body as getting run over by a bus. Your body does not know the difference. Surgery causes very acute pain. When the anesthesia wears off after a surgical procedure and a patient wakes up, his body enters the instinctive "fight or flight" mode. After all, pain is a warning system, alerting his body that something is wrong. After surgery, his body tries to assess what has gone wrong, and how best to fix it. In the stressful response, the gut slows down and the heart speeds up, causing, among other things, increased blood pressure and a total shutdown of the digestive system. These symptoms aggravate the healing process for a patient who has just had surgery. When surgical pain is properly managed, the patient not only feels better, but his entire body functions more normally and dedicates its energies to healing instead of panic.

The "fight or flight" response of the body is caused by the human hormone epinephrine, which is sometimes called adrenaline. In a stressful situation, extra epinephrine is released within the body, causing the heart to beat faster, preparing the body to defend itself. Some kinds of surgery (in the chest or upper abdominal area) might affect the lungs by preventing them from being fully expanded. This chest scar pain stops the patient from taking deep breaths, which, in turn, might cause part of a lung to collapse. This is called splinting, and it makes it difficult for a patient to breathe, and makes the patient vulnerable to pneumonia. Since the stress response has already taxed the patient's normal capacity to fight infection, pneumonia would obviously add an even greater burden to the recovery process.

As I mentioned earlier, most gut functions will shut down no matter where the surgery is because of the "fight or flight" response. Epinephrine takes blood flow away from the digestive system, dedicating extra blood flow to the arms and legs in order to confront the stressful situation. Until the gut is working normally, food and medications for post-op patients are usually delivered intravenously. And the patient can't leave the hospital until he is off all intravenous delivery systems for food and medications.

To top it off, a patient suffering from postop pain will very likely feel as if he's lost control over his own body and if the post-op pain is poorly managed, he might feel as if he is begging for more and more pain medications. With this sense of helplessness, in addition to the normal pain, a patient might easily fall into a state of depression.

Not only must I take these side effects into account

when treating a post-op pain patient, but I must also calcu-
late the wide variation of pain severity during the several
days following an operation. The degree of pain changes
considerably—from simple recovery and scar healing to
activities like sitting up, changing dressings, walking, and
so forth. A pain-management specialist must know to use a
pain medication that can accommodate this changing
dynamic.

Right after surgery, the one that most closely fits the bill
is a narcotic, such as morphine. Almost every surgery is followed by a narcotic pain reliever, usually administered as
an injection or in an IV, since the digestive tract is temporarily out of commission. The narcotics are very sedating, however, and when they're working at their peak, the
patient is usually very sleepy. Narcotics are most effective in
treating the widely varying degrees of post-op pain, but
even they present challenges for properly controlling pain.
Doctors usually write static doses of pain-relieving medications, and such a dose is often not adequate enough immediately after the surgery. Then, two days later, the same
dose is far too much. A day or two after that, the patient's
state has improved, and that same narcotics dose is now far
too much. The patient has gone from not being medicated
enough to being greatly overmedicated. Also, there is no
way to increase the medication to coincide with more
painful moments of activity, like standing or walking. The
patient's renewed discomfort on this occasion might
prompt her to call a nurse, who must then consult the doctor to determine whether more medication is needed. The
whole cycle takes time, from twenty minutes to an hour,
which can add to a patient's sense of helplessness.

There are a variety of new options to deliver narcotics safely and with much greater pain-relieving effects. One of them is the patient-controlled analgesic (PCA) device. Some patients are familiar with this "button" device used in hospitals, because it's been around for a couple of years. This allows the patient to control the dosage of the medication, within limits. The pain medication is connected to a patient's intravenous line, with a button-controlled device that is left in the patient's control. Parameters are set in advance that automatically control the amount of each dose, the time lapse between doses, the total amount per hour, and the total amount of medication per twenty-four hours. Beyond that, the patient can determine when he needs more medication, without calling a nurse. We know that an intravenous narcotic will reach peak effect in about eight minutes. No matter how many times he presses the button, the device will lock out for eight minutes at a time, between doses. There is a built-in limit that prevents the delivery of too much pain reliever, but it can permit the patient to use more when he needs it. By using smaller, more frequent doses of pain medication, the patient can adjust the pain control to corresponding activity levels. This not only relieves the pain more effectively, letting the patient get the doses when he needs it, but it gives him a greater sense of control.

Of course, the PCA can only be used intravenously, and only when the patient is able to understand its purpose and is capable of dosing himself. Other types of pain relief for post-op pain include epidural injections. Most pain receptors for narcotics are in the spinal column. Administering narcotics directly to the epidural space through an injection allows the receptors to feel pain relief without spreading narcotics throughout the body's whole system. It also requires much smaller doses, because the narcotic enters directly into the space around the spine and is not disseminated in other parts of the body.

In cases where ongoing relief is needed, a catheter might be inserted into the epidural space. This infusion can remain in place for several days, offering continuous pain medication after surgery. We call this procedure a central access delivery system. There are even such devices that allow the patient to control the dosage, similar to the PCA device. We frequently add a diluted anesthetic into the narcotic, allowing for a smaller amount of each medication, to combine their effects more potently than either of them alone. Sometimes the stomach functions return more quickly when the epidural catheter is used, and that's a good thing for the healing process. As you might imagine, however, the central access delivery infusions require well-trained hospital personnel to maintain.

Localized injections of simple anesthetics are also helpful with post-op pain. In cases of orthopedic surgeries, where bony pain might ensue, we use an injection of Toradol, which is a nonsteroidal anti-inflammatory medication, along with a narcotic. Toradol is the only non-steroidal anti-inflammatory that is available in an injectable format and approved by the Federal Drug Administration. When it is used in combination, Toradol enhances the effects of the narcotic, requiring a much lower dose of each.

More than that, there are new methods that can be used in advance of the surgery to lessen the severity of post-op pain. This is called preemptive analgesia, and it works virtual miracles with surgery, where the pain of incision is frequently the worst part of the procedure. This means delivering pain reliever, such as morphine, to a patient prior to surgery. It actually prevents the pain from getting very advanced later on, during and after surgery. This not only provides better pain relief, but its effects help the patient to recover at lightning speed.

When the patient's digestive system is back on track, and he is able to go home, we will switch to appropriate oral medications to keep the pain under control. And, of course, we supervise a proper physical therapy program to make sure the pain does not linger. With these innovative and anticipatory pain relief treatments, post-op pain should soon become a distant memory in the annals of health care.

SCIATICA

See Back Pain with Radiation.

SHINGLES

See Herpes Zoster.

SPINAL STENOSIS

See Back Pain with Radiation.

SPORTS INJURY

See Traumatic Injury.

TEMPOROMANDIBULAR JOINT DISORDER (TMJ) PAIN

Pain from the temporomandibular joint falls into the category of temporomandibular disorders (TMD). This includes pain in the joint and in the muscle around the joint, at the connection of the jaw. This is a localized pain related to a poor alignment of the joint and the mastication (chewing) muscle. It can also cause pain in the form of neck aches and toothaches. It is a fairly prevalent condition—one study estimated that as many as 14 percent of all adults suffer from TMJ pain.

The pain might follow an injury to the area, or a sudden change in the way the jaw is used while chewing. It can also be caused by a response to stress, to whiplash, or by a patient's clenching or grinding his teeth so much that the jaw becomes realigned. TMJ pain hurts while one is talking and particularly when one is eating. In fact, these activities might become intolerably painful, causing the patient to modify his chewing or talking, which makes the condition even worse. The pain might recede if the jaw is not being used, but it comes right back whenever the patient starts talking or eating.

The most effective treatment is aimed at finding out what's causing the poor alignment and addressing that problem, whether it be an injury or stress that's making the patient clench his jaw. Treatment sometimes involves a prosthetic device to return the jaw to normal alignment. The pain can be relieved with anti-inflammatories, combined with a muscle relaxant. This allows the muscles to relax and the patient to get a good night's sleep. Sometimes, if the chewing muscle is in a spasm mode, it can be relieved with a trigger-point steroid injection.

Physical therapy is very important for strengthening the joint. And if someone is grinding her teeth, psychological counseling is very helpful. Conquering TMJ pain requires a concerted effort on behalf of the patient. Unlike many syndromes, TMJ often involves nearly every aspect of pain types and treatments.

TENDINITIS

This is swelling of the tissue that connects a muscle to a bone. When the tendons are inflamed, the pain is usually restricted to the afflicted area, and it is very sensitive to the touch. Sometimes it feels warm and swollen. This can be caused by chronic overuse of the tendon, or by simply overstretching it in a single incident. Tendons are not designed to be stretched the way a muscle is. When some patients discover they only hurt when the afflicted tendon is used, they simply stop moving it. If you don't move your arm, you might be able to pretend there isn't a problem with it. But that is a fairly intrusive form of pain management! The best thing to do is to reduce the inflammation with a nonsteroidal anti-inflammatory, and also by using alternate cold and hot compresses. Tendinitis is frequently cured by acupuncture.

When the swelling is reduced, it is important to retrain the tendon with physical therapy. If the tendon is not retrained to its proper memory, the tendinitis will simply return.

TERMINAL ILLNESS

See chapter 9.

TRAUMATIC INJURY

A traumatic injury covers a wide range of painful events, from a broken leg to emergency surgery, a deep cut, or internal bruising. It is usually a surprise event that involves a lot of pain for which no one is prepared.

One of the most frustrating elements of traumatic pain is that the patient is frequently treated by doctors she doesn't know, in a strange hospital, perhaps, and at the mercy of an unknown health-care system. After she is discharged, she may have no idea where to go for rehabilitation, and no time to research in advance the various available treatments. If it weren't for these overwhelming factors, treatment of a traumatic pain would be similar to that of postoperative pain. But the emergency setting makes traumatic injury pain a special syndrome, because in addition to the pain itself are the natural consequences of being unprepared.

As with a scheduled surgery, a traumatic event causes the body to go into the hormonal "fight or flight" response. The difference with trauma is that the injury is not predictable or localized. There is no preparatory time prior to a traumatic injury, no time for diagnostic tests or medication adjustments. Not only is traumatic injury unpredictable, but it frequently involves multiple areas of the body that need repair. One injury might inhibit the healing process of another. After a bicycle accident, Mike B. could not do the rehabilitative exercises for his injured back, because he also had a fractured leg. His improper gait with the leg cast made his injured back even worse. The individual injuries were then compounded by frustration and stress.

The pain management for traumatic injury is similar to that for post-op patients. The treatment is very individualized to the injuries, naturally. But our goal is to get the patient back to normal functions, including those parts that are in pain. By using local nonsteroidal anti-inflammatories, local anesthetics, or narcotics, the pain should be treated to the point where it has no negative effects on the patient. Realistic goals for recovery should be set, permitting the use of these pain relievers to keep pain and stress at low levels. It usually takes more time to recover from the pain of traumatic injury than from the trauma itself, whether the ailment is a minor surgery or a kidney stone. A doctor's rule of thumb is that for every day a patient remains injured, three days will be required for recovery. If Jill A. gets hit by a car and is hospitalized for a month, it will take three months of rehabilitation for her to return to normal functioning. The earlier the rehabilitation can begin with realistic goals, the faster a patient's recovery will be.

We find that most traumatic pain patients have a great desire to recover, and this also speeds the healing process.

TRIGEMINAL NEURALGIA

This is a type of nerve pain that afflicts the major nerve in the face. The pain of the trigeminal nerve can be excruciating, and its cause is not known, although it is frequently associated with trauma such as a car accident. Attacks may occur every few minutes for days, or even weeks. The nerve pain can trigger muscle spasms in the face as well.

The best treatment for trigeminal neuralgia is a nonsteroidal anti-inflammatory along with an anticonvulsant such as Neurontin. Nerve block injections of the trigeminal nerve with a local anesthetic and steroid can also be helpful. Over time, this ailment might disappear, and the medications can be stopped. It is advisable to keep the medications on hand, however, in the event you feel an attack coming on. Prevention is always easier and more effective that pain treatment! In certain cases where medications cannot be used, a patient might obtain permanent relief with a radiofrequency ablation of the trigeminal nerve, as described in chapter 8. For trigeminal neuralgia, it is imperative to consult a neurologist or a pain-management specialist.

VASCULAR PAIN

Vascular pain is usually chronic pain in the feet or up into the legs. It is caused by decreased blood flow. Vascular pain is common in the elderly, whose arteries are simply narrowing with age, inhibiting the flow of blood to extremities like the arms and legs. As with diabetic polyneuropathy, I have found that antiarrhythmic heart medications like Mexitil (mexiletine) work well for vascular pain. I complement this treatment by prescribing regular exercise in a warm environment, to facilitate increased blood flow. Your primary health-care provider should be able to treat your vascular pain successfully. If nothing else helps, then you might consider spinal cord stimulation, as discussed in chapter 8. This technique increases the capacity of small blood vessels to carry oxygen to tissues.

These are the primary syndromes of my pain-management practice. If you have a diagnosis that does not appear here, work with your doctor to determine which of the six pain types from chapter 2 comprise your particular syndrome. No matter what is causing your pain condition, a combination of medications can make you pain-free and allow you to begin physical therapy. It helps to know the name of your pain syndrome, but there are some cases I treat that defy such classification. That does not mean we cannot successfully break down its parts and eliminate the pain.

In rare cases, pain syndromes must be treated with procedures such as surgery that are beyond the four-step Painbuster program. I call these techniques "advanced procedures," and they are explained in chapter 8.

The following chart encapsulates the most successful elements of initial therapies for the pain of these diseases. It is arranged so you can see the variety of pain types and why combinations of treatment are necessary.

Disease	Nerve	Visceral	Myofascial	Bony	Sympathetic	Psychogenic	Other
Abdominal Pain		•tricyclic antidepressant	•trigger-point injection		•nerve block injection	•counseling	
Ankylosing Spondylitis				•acupuncture •NSAID rotation •trigger-point injection			
Arthritis				•NSAID rotation			•glucosamine chondroitin
Back Pain (myofascial)	•tricyclic antidepressant		•acupuncture •muscle relaxants •NSAID before bedtime •trigger-point injection			•stress counseling	•hot and cold packs •TENS
Back Pain with Radiation	•tricyclic antidepressant •epidural steroid injection		•NSAID	•trigger-point injection		•stress counseling	•surgery might be necessary

Disease	Nerve	Visceral	Myofascial	Bony	Sympathetic	Psychogenic	Other
Bursitis				• heat packs • NSAID			
Cancer	• lidocaine patch • tricyclic antidepressant	• nerve block injection	• acupuncture • narcotics	• NSAID or aspirin • narcotics	• nerve block injection	• counseling	• intrathecal infusion
Carpal Tunnel Syndrome			• acupuncture • trigger-point injection				
Central Pain Syndrome	• Neurontin • tricyclic antidepressant • narcotics			• NSAID or aspirin			
CRPS, Type I					• acupuncture • sympathetic nerve block injection • epidural catheter • bretylium bier blockade • SCS		• surgically repair damaged nerve

Disease	Nerve	Visceral	Myofascial	Bony	Sympathetic	Psychogenic	Other
CRPS, Type II					• acupuncture • sympathetic nerve block injection • epidural catheter • bretylium bier blockade • SCS	• stress counseling	
Diabetic Polyneuropathy	• cardiac antiarrhythmic • NSAID						
Fibromyalgia			• acupuncture • muscle relaxant • NSAID	• NSAID • trigger-point injection		• group therapy	• biofeedback
Gout				• NSAID • narcotics			• treat cause of inflammation
Herpes Zoster and Postherpetic Neuralgia	• tricyclic antidepressant • NSAID • epidural steroid injection						• antiviral medication

Disease	Nerve	Visceral	Myofascial	Bony	Sympathetic	Psychogenic	Other
HIV	• tricyclic antidepressant	• narcotics	• NSAID		• acupuncture	• psychological counseling	
Intercostal Neuritis	• tricyclic antidepressant • nerve block injection						• ablation
Obstetric Pain		• acupuncture • narcotics • epidural injection of local anesthetic and narcotics					• breathing techniques
Pelvic Pain	• tricyclic antidepressant • nerve block injection		• psychological counseling • narcotics		• nerve block injection	• counseling	
Phantom Limb Pain	• tricyclic antidepressant • SCS • epidural infusion					• counseling	

Disease	Nerve	Visceral	Myofascial	Bony	Sympathetic	Psychogenic	Other
Post-op Pain	• tricyclic antidepressant		• acupuncture • narcotics • NSAID				• preemptive analgesia
TMJ			• NSAID • trigger-point injection • muscle relaxant				• repair jaw alignment
Tendinitis			• NSAID • acupuncture				• hot and cold packs
Traumatic Injury	• narcotics	• nerve block injection	• NSAID • narcotics	• NSAID	• nerve block injection	• counseling	
Trigeminal Neuralgia	• acupuncture • NSAID • anticonvulsant medication						
Vascular Pain			• antiarrhythmic medications				

CHAPTER 8

Advanced Procedures and Surgery

T here are some pain cases where the most effective long-term treatment is not just exercise and proper diet, but continued medication or regular injections on a periodic basis. A patient who has spinal stenosis, for example, might need to have an epidural steroid injection every eight months, for the rest of his life. A periodic epidural injection may be the most effective, convenient, and least invasive option to control his chronic pain. I believe that is preferable treatment to an irreversible procedure or invasive surgery. I always prefer the least invasive techniques— medication or injection therapy—and I achieve successful pain relief without surgery for nearly every patient who comes into my office. A small percentage, however, fewer than 20 percent of my patients, are not cured using noninvasive methods. Fortunately, there are a number of other techniques that help even the most incapacitated chronic pain patients.

I recommend each of these as a last resort—some of these methods are not reversible, so even accounting for the risks of side effects, they must offer a greater benefit than if they were not used. And these must be administered by an experienced practitioner. Many of these techniques are used in combination with the traditional Painbuster maintenance program. If one of these advanced procedures can control your pain, I prefer that you consider this rather than continuing to live in chronic pain. Almost anything is better than that. And, often, some of these procedures preclude the need for additional medications or ongoing treatments. So even though I recommend these as a last resort, and they are not an element of my traditional Painbuster program, these procedures can be very effective.

LIDOCAINE INFUSION THERAPY

This technique is simply a periodic intravenous infusion of a local anesthetic, and it can be very helpful in reducing a variety of nerve pains. It is most commonly used for those who suffer from diabetic polyneuropathy, or patients who have widespread pain in small nerve fibers. Doctors believe that lidocaine infusion therapy—which has been used since the 1940s—decreases the transmission of pain impulses before they reach the spinal cord. The infusion requires an intravenous line with a dose of lidocaine in the IV solution. Pain relief begins almost immediately and remains effective for several weeks afterward. This is a noninvasive procedure that is commonly used across the country, but it does require between three and eight hours of treatment at a doctor's office or hospital, once a week.

Some doctors use an infusion of phentolamine instead of a local anesthetic. This is a potent drug that expands the blood vessels and increases blood flow to areas where it is weak.

I have found that newer oral medications, such as mexiletine, achieve similar relief for nerve pain, without the hassle or expense of frequent office visits. If you have nerve pain that is not alleviated by any other medication therapy, or you prefer the use of an IV so that your medication doses are smaller and not disseminated through your digestive system, then you might want to consider lidocaine infusion.

PROLOTHERAPY

Prolotherapy is also called proliferative therapy or ligament reconstructive therapy. This is a reversible procedure that has existed, in various rudimentary forms, for hundreds of years. In the 1920s, a physician named George Hackett refined its modern technique, which is often the best way to alleviate pain caused by damaged tendons and ligaments, or muscle disorders.

Muscles are not directly attached to bones. They are linked to bones by ligaments and tendons. Muscles were designed to be stretched, within limits, and then to return to normal size after any exertion. Tendons and ligaments were not designed to be stretched at all. When a bone needs to be moved, your muscles do all the necessary stretching for everything. If a ligament or a tendon is forced to stretch, however, such as in a traumatic injury, it will frequently remain stretched, unable to return to normal. In a car accident, sometimes a person's neck ligaments might be stretched, causing pain that is commonly known as whiplash. If you stretch out your arms to catch a heavy falling object, you would cause a similar injury to your elbow.

The pain is being caused by nerves passing through the ligament into the muscle. Since the ligament was stretched, its nerves have also been traumatized and pulled beyond normal capacity. In addition, the adjacent muscle senses that the normal ligament tension is gone, and it pulls harder to make up for the slack. This can bring on a painful muscle spasm, on top of the ligament pain.

When pain is being generated by a stretched ligament or tendon, prolotherapy is used to tighten these structures. This repair is not always easy, because ligaments and tendons do not grow much, and they do not have a lot of blood flow. Prolotherapy uses an injection to irritate the tendon or ligament, forcing it to become larger so the slackness disappears. As the swelling recedes, sometimes the tendon shrinks back down to normal size, and the pain goes away. It doesn't always work, but because it is relatively noninvasive, it is worth trying.

The injection delivers any number of substances into the tendon, at various points, with a small needle. The injection might be a concentrated glucose solution, pumice, sodium morrhuate (a derivation of cod-liver oil), and a fluid called P2G, which is a combination of lidocaine, glucose, glycerin, and phenol (a chemical derivative of coal tar). It takes a few days for prolotherapy to have any effect—the inflammation has to subside before we can see if the injection manipulated the tendon or ligament back to its healthy state. The procedure can be safely repeated, if necessary.

Physical therapy is a vital adjunct to prolotherapy. Without strengthening the injured area during the pain relief, it is certain to be injured again.

NEUROABLATION

A neuroablation is one of several procedures that destroys a sensory nerve or muscle tissue in order to eliminate pain. This is as irreversible as it sounds, which is one reason why I resort to this technique only after all others have failed. Some nerves can regenerate themselves—that is, they grow back after being destroyed—but many do not. The goal is that a new nerve will grow and it will no longer be painful. Alternatively, patients should understand that a new nerve might not appear, in which case the area might feel "different," but it should no longer feel pain.

There are three basic methods of neuroablation, which are usually determined by whichever one your doctor prefers. Each achieves essentially the same result. Before any of them are used, however, I begin by injecting a local anesthetic into the target area. This numbs the spot for a couple of hours, and then it returns to normal. If the temporary injection brings relief, then we know a neuroablation will achieve this positive effect permanently. Not only will this local injection predict whether the permanent ablation will bring pain relief, it will also indicate to the patient what the side effects might feel like. The numbing effect will not only relieve the pain, it will change the feeling in the nerve and also in the entire area served by that nerve. For example, if a patient with intercostal nerve pain from a fractured rib gets an ablation of the intercostal nerve, the senses around the entire nerve—and the rib—will be numbed permanently. Under local anesthetic, the patient might not be able to feel his rib cage expanding and contracting with each normal breath, and he may not like that sensation. His actual breathing is not affected, but the patient may find the numbness is not comfortable. The local anesthetic injection allows the patient to get an idea of what a neuroablation will feel like before he decides to have the change made permanently. The patient must decide if this feeling is acceptable and preferable to the nerve pain. If so, then one of the following three types of neuroablation may work very well to resolve his pain syndrome.

Cryoablation

Sometimes a sensory nerve is destroyed by freezing it. A needlelike instrument uses compressed gas to make the tip as cold as minus seventy (−70) degrees Celsius, which is cold enough to kill a nerve. Only the tip is cold, not the rest of the needle. Depending on the size of the tip, cryoablation can freeze as much as five millimeters of nerve or tissue. It is very focused, for precise treatment of small areas. An ice crystal forms inside the nerve, destroying it, but the surrounding "architecture" remains intact. This means the nerve might slowly grow back in the same space. The track of the old nerve is maintained, and it usually has time to "reset" itself to a pain-free status before the new nerve grows in. It is hoped that this nerve will not be painful. Everything around it is normal, so there is every chance that the nerve will grow in painlessly. Sometimes, nerve growth forms a tangled cluster (what is known as a neuroma) instead of a normal nerve. A neuroma can cause new pain all its own. With cryoablation, however, the likelihood of neuroma is not great.

A preliminary test with a local anesthetic ensures the proper placement of the permanent freezing probe. The cryoablation procedure takes only a few minutes. The chronic pain should be gone immediately, replaced perhaps by a dull ache, which might last as long as a week. After that, all pain should be gone for good. The damaged nerve will take between three and nine months to grow back, by which time your body has recovered from whatever was causing the pain there. Sometimes, after several months, the new nerve grows back with a small amount of pain. If the procedure is repeated, I find that the nerve will have diminished pain each time, until it is finally gone altogether.

Radio-Frequency Ablation

Radio-frequency ablation (RF) achieves the same effect as cryoablation, except it uses heat to destroy nerves instead of freezing them. The heat is generated by a very high frequency radio wave, which is transmitted to the tip of the needle. This heat will generally destroy about three millimeters of tissue, so RF is even more precise than a freezing probe. This procedure is considered more permanent than cryoablation, because a new nerve is less likely to grow back after an RF ablation. That means the pain won't come back either. However, this procedure has a greater chance of neuroma, the formation of a sometimes painful nerve mass. RF ablation is particularly effective for patients who have facet joint pain that is not relieved with injections or medications.

Patients find this procedure slightly more painful than cryoablation, and recovery takes a few days longer. Other than that, these procedures are very similar and usually selected based on your doctor's preference and experience. Both RF and cryoablation are relatively precise techniques, perfect for treating a single, small nerve. For larger areas, we turn to a special kind of injection.

Alcohol or Phenol Injection

This is an injectable ablation that has been used for a very long time, before the days of RF or cryoablation. While RF and cryoablation allow for a more precise target area— smaller than five millimeters—these injections permanently destroy tissue wherever the fluid spreads. We call this area the kill zone. These injections also eliminate the architecture, making it virtually impossible for nerves to grow back in this area. This method requires only a simple needle to perform, to inject alcohol or phenol into the epidural space.

These injections are reserved for cases where larger areas need to be destroyed. One example would be a patient who has chronic pain from pancreatic cancer. The celiac plexus is a large nerve cluster bundled around the aorta in the center of the abdomen. This plexus is about five inches in diameter. If we tried to alleviate the patient's nerve pain with an RF or cryoablation, we would have to spend many hours moving the tiny probe to cover such a large area, millimeter by millimeter. But an injection would cover the entire area in a single procedure and would be considered the more appropriate way to go.

Neuroablations are very effective, and their risks of side effects are very low. If you are one of the few who have nerve pain that lingers after using the Painbuster program, then this alternative is a good one for you.

BOTOX INJECTION

Botox is short for botulinum toxin, and if it sounds a lot like botulism poisoning, there is good reason for that. Botox, as used in a pain-relieving injection, is the same bacterium that sometimes infiltrates food products and causes food poisoning. It is toxic, but this bacterium is a long-acting muscle relaxant. It can be used for trigger-point injections into small muscles that are spasming and causing pain. This is similar to a trigger-point injection using a local anesthetic, only the Botox lasts much longer. Sometimes, it will paralyze the muscle forever. Because of the risks of the Botox spreading to healthy areas and caus-ing widespread muscle weakness, I do not recommend these injections for my patients. I have known people whose pain was relieved using this technique, but I prefer more reliable, reversible, and less toxic procedures for muscle spasm.

Surgically Implanted Devices for Pain Control

Most patients with chronic pain find a resolution with one of the nonsurgical methods we have reviewed thus far. However, there are a handful of patients who reach this level of care for relieving their pain syndromes, because everything else has failed. You might be saying to yourself, every time this doctor describes a new pain-management technique, he begins by saying "when all else has failed." Perhaps it sounds as if my Painbuster program has a large number of failures. But it doesn't. Eighty percent of my patients are cured of chronic pain without any advanced procedure or surgery. But for that small percentage who are still in pain, I postpone advanced techniques, including surgery, not only because the risks are high, but because we might harm the body's natural design. If the advanced procedure is not effective, we may have also destroyed any chances for your body to go back and respond to a less invasive option.

The following techniques offer very potent pain management and, for some patients, they offer the only solution for pain control. These require special training to implement them, as well as enough experience to understand the goal of this therapy. Not all physicians practicing pain management are trained in these procedures, but you should be able to locate one without difficulty, no matter where you live.

EPIDURAL CATHETER

There are many surgical procedures performed by pain-management specialists who are also anesthesiologists, orthopedic surgeons, or neurosurgeons. Probably the most common procedure performed by these specialists is the placement of an epidural catheter, a tube that delivers medication into the epidural space. The goal is to send pain meds to the area right next to the nerves responsible for the pain. This is ideal for a patient who will need the pain medication for two months or less, such as someone with a traumatic injury. It is similar to intrathecal infusion, except this pump is external, and about the size of a Walkman, which is easily refilled with medication. The side effects that are associated with oral medications are almost nonexistent with the catheter. This permits medication of a chronic pain while using a minimum dose, and most patients experience excellent pain relief.

INTRADISCAL ELECTROTHERMAL THERAPY

In the mid-1990s, researchers discovered that some chronic lower back pain comes from spontaneous disintegration of the disc itself. This is called pain with a "discogenic" origin and is quite different from a herniated disc. With this disease, cracks form on the outside wall of the disc and the goopy interior begins to leak through. Since the structure of the disc also contains tiny nerve fibers that feel pain, this causes an additional pain, aside from the adjacent nerve and muscular pain. A simple test where dye is injected into the disc will reveal this condition. It is a permanent condition, as the cracks will not repair themselves. Intradiscal electrothermal therapy is the best solution, and it is quite painless. A needle is inserted through the patient's back into the disc. Next, an electrode is inserted through the needle and threaded through the interior of the disc. When it is in the proper place, the electrode is heated in order to harden the disc, filling in any defects and preventing further deterioration of the disc. It serves as a permanent "spackle" for the cracks, and it can greatly alleviate chronic discogenic pain.

SPINAL CORD STIMULATION

This pain relief method was first devised in the 1950s, when it was known as dorsal column stimulation. Spinal cord stimulation (SCS) is a surgical technique that places electrodes in the epidural space, at the level where the nerve roots converge. If there is chronic nerve pain in the legs, for instance, we would place the electrodes in the lower spinal area where the leg nerves enter the spinal cord. When a low current is run through the electrodes, it stimulates the spinal cord, replacing the sensation of pain with a sensation of slight vibration. The concept is very similar to TENS, except in this treatment the current stimulates nerves instead of muscles. As with many pain relief techniques, it is not completely known why this electrical current obliterates pain, although there are many theories.

In the 1960s, SCS required surgery through the bones of the spine to implant electrical wires in the body. Current techniques are less invasive, with percutaneous (through the skin) placement of electrical leads, although the patient is still sedated. SCS is best used for patients who have nerve pain from radiculopathy, but who have found only temporary relief with epidural steroid injections. Other good candidates for SCS are people with postherpetic neuralgia, phantom limb pain, or complex regional pain syndrome (CRPS), who respond only temporarily to sympathetic nerve block injections using local anesthetics. These patients have shown a response to treatment, but only on a temporary basis; they need something that lasts longer than an injection. SCS has the same pain-relieving effects as a local block, but on a permanent basis. If all the other noninvasive options are tested and not successful in controlling pain, then I feel that SCS is a good alternative to consider.

I also believe it is imperative to obtain psychological counseling before SCS implantation, for two reasons. The first is to determine how the patient might respond once the SCS removes all his pain. Believe it or not, this void might be difficult for a long-term pain patient to handle. The patient might even subconsciously replace the SCS-cured pain with something else—perhaps, even, a new pain. I have seen this happen more than once. I had a patient, Midge D., who had tried everything for her severe lumbar radiculopathy. We finally implanted a spinal cord stimulator, and her pain disappeared almost overnight. She was amazed, because she hadn't been without pain for about eight years. She even liked the new vibrating sensation. After only a week, however, she developed a new pain in her abdomen. It was obviously not related to the radiculopathy, which had been completely resolved with the SCS. I was at a loss to explain the origins of her new pain. Eventually, Midge became incapacitated by this new pain, for which we could find absolutely no cause. She is still seeing a psychologist to try to resolve this new pain. Her radiculopathy, on the other hand, has not resurfaced since she got the SCS. Sometimes I wonder if the new pain wasn't caused by the resolution of the original pain. Counseling helps some patients put painlessness into perspective.

The second reason for psychological evaluation is to help determine if the patient would accept the use of a "mechanical" technology to control his pain. Some studies have shown that if certain patients are not comfortable being connected to a battery-operated device, however small and unobtrusive, their bodies will reject its good effects. Even if the electrical stimulation is the best relief a patient has felt in years, their discomfort with "alien technology" can cause their bodies to work against it.

Good communication is another vital element to the success of this technique. Prior to SCS, the patient and the doctor must make clear to each other the exact area that needs to be treated, and what their expectations are. After all, a seventy-year-old man who gets an SCS implanted, after years of chronic pain, will not emerge from the procedure as a youthful Olympic athlete. It is often helpful to have a trial implantation, using an external receiver attached to the percutaneous leads. The stimulator should replace the pain with a vibrating sensation, which many patients describe as pleasurable. The test period might last a few days or as long as a month, after which the patient can determine whether to implant a permanent SCS device. If the temporary device has no effect, then you know the permanent one won't either. If it works well, however, then so will the permanent device, which is a small receiver placed under the skin with a minor surgical procedure. Small adjustments to the device can be made after it is implanted, to fine-tune the stimulation for optimal pain relief.

As with all Painbuster treatments, after pain relief is achieved using SCS, the patient undergoes extensive rehabilitation to return her body to normal functionality. Since the SCS patient typically has had pain for a very long time, physical therapy can take several months. And, of course, the maintenance program lasts a lifetime.

INTRATHECAL INFUSION DEVICE

As discussed in chapter 5, this is one of the most effective ways to deliver pain medications to the fluid around the spinal cord. It offers the highest concentration of medication where it needs to be, using the minimal dose. The intrathecal infusion device is a delivery system that is best used when the side effects of oral medications are too overwhelming for a patient. The medications may be working, but there are simply too many other problems; poor combinations with the other drugs being used to treat the disease, perhaps, or severe intolerance in the digestive system.

This device, which is the size of a hockey puck, is surgically implanted in a patient's abdomen, with a tiny tube that delivers the medication directly to the subarachnoid fluid around the spinal cord, where the pain receptors are. It serves as sort of an internal pump, which can be refilled in a doctor's office every few months. This concept is similar to the epidural catheter, only this one is designed for someone who needs long-term medication for chronic pain relief.

There are several types of medication that are traditionally used in an intrathecal infusion device: narcotics (usually morphine) and muscle relaxants (primarily Baclofen), among others. Medication treatment with this pump requires about one hundredth, or even one thousandth, of the dose used in oral form. This smaller amount has the same pain-relieving power of larger oral doses, with fewer side effects because the intrathecal dose is so low. The intrathecal infusion pump provides steady, long-lasting pain relief. Unlike SCS, this pump may require dosage adjustment over time, and it needs to be refilled on a regular basis. The doctor simply places a needle through the skin and into the device, filling it with a new supply of medication.

As with SCS, noninvasive treatments should be explored before implanting this device. If the side effects from traditional oral medications outweigh the benefits, then the patient should undergo psychological counseling to determine if she is a good candidate for an intrathecal infusion pump. Also, a test must be administered to ensure that medication in the epidural space has the desired effect. A temporary catheter into the epidural space can deliver the same medication. During its use the patient can determine if the permanent pump will be effective. If the test does not bring pain relief to the patient, then it is unlikely the pump will—some patients do not respond to this treatment. If this is the case, then an alternative, such as an ablation, should be pursued.

The implantation of an intrathecal infusion pump is a minor surgical procedure, but it usually requires a short stay at the hospital. The patient never feels the weight of the device, which remains completely under the skin, in the abdomen. The medication might be adjusted afterward, until pain relief is constant and comfortable. Of course, this is just the beginning of this patient's treatment: progressive physical therapy is required to bring the body back to normal pain-free function.

Surgery

As a rule, I do not recommend this aggressive and invasive therapy unless all other treatments have been ruled out. All surgery is an invasive procedure that always carries a risk of infection, and cutting damages a lot of healthy tissue along the way. Surgery is irreversible and, last but not least, surgery causes plenty of pain by itself. If there is a clear indication that surgery can reverse a painful situation, such as a broken bone or a herniated disc that is causing progressive weakness in the legs, then I recommend moving directly to this solution. In other cases, if more conservative medication therapy has failed to achieve pain relief, and it is clear from a CT or MRI that surgery is the best hope for resolving the problem, then surgery might be your next best step.

DISCECTOMY

There is a common debate regarding patients who have herniated discs as to whether surgery is preferable to medication management. My view is, if the pain can be eliminated by using nonsurgical techniques, such as epidural steroid injections, then those are preferable because they carry fewer risks than back surgery. However, there are cases where nonsurgical techniques are not an option at all. For example, if a herniated disc is causing progressive weakness in an arm or a leg, or if it is pushing on a nerve that affects normal function of the bowel or bladder, the patient needs immediate surgery to remove the extruding disc. The pressure needs to be removed from the nerve before there is permanent damage. This condition may not even present itself as pain; the patient might feel numbness or weakness in the areas served by the nerve that is being bumped by the disc. In these cases, there is no question that surgery is the only way to resolve the problem. When I see a patient whose arm or leg is getting progressively weaker, and her MRI shows a herniated disc hitting on a nerve, I might tell her, "You need surgery, as soon as possible."

If pain is the primary symptom of a herniated disc, then most cases—four out of every five patients—can be successfully treated with medications and injections, which do not carry the usual risks of surgery. Pressure on the painful nerve will be relieved while the disc heals itself, and we strengthen nearby muscles in the Painbuster program. If it is not absolutely necessary to have surgery, then I do not think any patient should have it. By the same token, if injections and medications are not helping to reduce the pain from a herniated disc, then surgery should be considered. Long-term inflammation of the nerve can cause permanent damage. A discectomy, of course, means the patient must be treated with post-op pain management as well. Whatever treatment is taken, both must be followed by rehabilitation. Physical therapy prevents the same problem from recurring.

One other disease that responds well to surgery for pain relief is cancer. If a growth or tumor is pressing on tissue and is causing pain, then the pain is best erased by directly eliminating the pressure. In some cases, this might be surgical removal of the tumor. Of course, the doctor and patient must consider the overall condition of the patient and the risk of surgery. With advanced cases, such surgery would not serve to cure the disease itself, but merely to alleviate pain. Surgery can also help reduce the amount of pain medications needed for a cancer patient.

SPINAL FUSION

I am not a proponent of spinal fusion, mostly because I have seen many pain patients who were not helped by it. But there are cases where spinal fusion is very effective. If there is an instability of the bones in the spine, caused by degenerative weakness or severe injury, the operation fuses two or more vertebrae together permanently. This sort of inflexible "bridge" halts painful movement in the area and connects the healthy vertebrae on either side. The structure of the spine remains intact and flexible, except for the small area where the fusion holds the bones rigid. The materials used to connect the bones range from titanium screws and intricate springs to bone fragments taken from the patient's pelvis.

With a successful fusion, you can hardly detect any change in the patient's spine appearance and natural motion. Because of the nature of my work, however, I see a lot of patients who have had spinal fusion, yet they still have the same pain they had before the surgery. And now the pain is in an area that has permanently limited motion. Not only that, but the fusion itself frequently causes another type of pain, such as when a small screw presses against a nerve.

Treating pain from a failed back surgery is a large part of my practice. If you have damaged vertebrae, or progressively worsening weakness in your spine—a hereditary trait, perhaps—then this surgery can stop the damage. But if your primary symptom is pain, and you want to treat the pain, then I would recommend other techniques.

NEURECTOMY AND SYMPATHECTOMY

A common procedure is the surgical destruction of a nerve by cutting it, so the pain loop is physically "interrupted." If the nerve is large enough, and easily reached through surgery, then sometimes this is better than a neuroablation. Cutting a sensory nerve is known as neurectomy; sympathectomy is the similar destruction of a sympathetic nerve. Being able to see the nerve during normal surgery allows for precise destruction of the proper nerve, so the success rate is high. Severe pain patients might even have a cordectomy, which is the removal of part of the spinal cord. A good candidate for surgical removal of a nerve is someone suffering from phantom limb pain who is not helped by less invasive methods such as nerve blocks. Doctor and patient should weigh the benefits carefully, but this is usually a very successful means to achieve relief from chronic pain.

While advanced procedures are best reserved for pain patients who have tried other options first, there is no doubt that, once you've reached this point, many of them are very effective. Some of these can be performed by a pain-management specialist such as myself, but not all of them. Since neurosurgery is not my specialty, I frequently refer discectomy patients, and those in need of other advanced procedures, to a neurosurgeon.

Do not go under the knife unless you understand every step of the surgical procedure and what its results will be. I have met new patients who tell me they've had back surgery for their pain syndrome, but they're not sure what, or why. And there they are, in my office, still in pain. If you are considering an advanced procedure to control your chronic pain, be sure it is one described in this book. I do not know of any others that can affect your pain, no matter what its cause.

CHAPTER 9

Dying without Pain:
Palliative Care for the Terminal Patient

Most of my patients are people who return to normal health and resume a highly functional life. Some of my patients, however, know that they will not return to good health. These patients need a special kind of pain management, where the priorities are adjusted on an individual basis, for each situation. You might think that this kind of pain management is the most straightforward and simple. But, in fact, it is the most difficult, because many such patients (and their doctors) still believe that death is the best cure for terminal pain.

I am always interested in legal arguments that surround the issue of doctor-assisted suicide. The extensive media coverage is surprising to me, not because this is a popular controversial issue, but because it never mentions other ways in which these patients might end a life of pain. It is not the Middle Ages; death is no longer the only cure for chronic pain. My personal belief is that a dying person and her doctor should never have to confront the issue of ending her life—not just from a legal standpoint but from a medical one. If the pain of a terminal patient is properly managed while maintaining her clarity of thought, would that patient still choose to hasten her death?

Like all my patients, a terminal patient deserves a lucid, satisfying life without pain. With modern pain relief medicine, euthanasia should no longer need to be an option to relieve the suffering of dying. I believe doctors who support euthanasia have the right intention—to provide relief for a patient in painful despair—but I prefer a pain-management regimen that doesn't serve merely to extend a human life but to extend the quality of that life.

There is a stigma attached to adequate pain relief, among patients, their families, and even their doctors. In this regard, the dying person is often the most neglected of patients. He hardly wants to spend his last weeks contradicting his doctor but, frequently, he is the only advocate for proper pain management at the end of his life.

The *Journal of the American Medical Association* reported in January 1999 that 50 percent of all patients who die in a hospital suffer severe pain that is not sufficiently treated. In cases where terminal cancer patients were over age sixty-five and in nursing homes, only 26 percent were given any pain medication at all. It is not surprising, then, that the process of dying is feared more than death itself. Of all the elements in health care, providing proper pain relief at the end of someone's life should be the most straightforward treatment to prescribe and administer. Seeking pain relief is a human biological instinct, and we now have dozens of ways to obtain it. Yet, even today, pain is one of the terminal patient's greatest fears, for it is still widely undertreated. I believe it is this fear, in addition to the pain itself, that drives patients to seek a premature death. Unrelieved pain has enormous psychological effects on all patients, but it is particularly catastrophic for a terminal patient, whose days are limited not only in quality but in quantity. A patient sometimes "catastrophizes," actually worsens her own pain, with this sense of hopelessness.

Inadequate pain management may sometimes result from subconscious undertreatment by doctors, who know that law enforcement officials are watchful over their narcotics prescriptions, particularly for terminal patients. In certain states, a doctor must use a special pad to prescribe narcotics to any patient. This pad makes three copies of the prescription: one for the doctor, one for the pharmacist, and another for the state drug enforcement agency. This pad is registered in chronological order, and its pages are closely monitored. In some cases, a doctor may subconsciously choose an alternative to narcotics because he wants to avoid government scrutiny. In other instances, patients have been undertreated for pain merely because the doctor did not have this triplicate prescription pad handy. The doctor might prescribe a weaker analgesic instead, perhaps even an ineffective or inappropriate one, because it can be written on a standard prescription pad.

A decade ago, there were no laws protecting doctors from prosecution for what seemed to be "mercy killing" by overmedication. But the explosion in medical advances to fight pain, as well as tireless efforts of researchers, the American Medical Association, and patient-support groups, have changed the attitudes of patients, doctors, and drug enforcement agencies. Within the last five years, nineteen states have enacted laws to protect doctors who prescribe pain medications to ailing patients, and a dozen more are considering such legislation. And some states have started to eliminate the triplicate requirement for narcotics prescriptions. In the meantime, however, the narcotics stigma has been insidiously embedded in the minds of doctors and patients over multiple generations.

Confronting the end of one's life is indescribable, by we who are in good health. We have read and studied much about the human stages of denial, anger, bargaining, depression, and acceptance in the face of death. Imagine having to do it all in a state of great pain, or in conflict with your health-care provider, or on a quest to bring on your demise even faster. No one's end should be so burdened.

Some doctors speak to me about their concerns for the "double effect" of pain medications. This is when the terminal patient becomes vulnerable to the side effects of pain-relieving narcotics, such as sedation or slower breathing (what doctors call respiratory depression). These patients may have their pain finally under control, for example, and then they die from respiratory depression. Are we then unintentionally causing their deaths, or perhaps even performing a "mercy killing" with narcotics? I believe the answer is, simply, no: we are merely treating their pain. It is not our goal to endanger the patient, and we are careful to monitor all medications. But if he dies, we know at least he will have done so in a pain-free state.

I once treated a sixty-seven-year-old terminal patient, Peter L., whose vital organs were slowly shutting down from a lifetime of severe hepatitis. He had also suffered several compound fractures ten years earlier and had been virtually immobilized by pain for years. Peter and I agreed that his pain management would never return him to the squash courts, but that it would be nice if he were not so distracted by his pain in his remaining months. I implanted an intrathecal infusion pump, which allowed Peter to function quite normally, and without pain. Three months later, Peter's wife came to see me. She said Peter's last weeks were the happiest he'd been in years, not necessarily because he was pain-free, but because he finally got a decent night's sleep. Pain had kept him awake for ten years. With intrathecal infusion, he slept so well that one morning he simply didn't wake up. Peter's wife wanted to thank me for helping to bring him peace at the end of his life, which had also brought some peace to her own.

That incident was a professional touchstone for me. I don't provide death as a pain relief option. I can offer a truly comfortable life to the living, for as long as they live. It may never be emotionally painless to confront death, but it can, at least, be physically painless. Here are some common misconceptions I encounter when I meet a dying patient who is in pain.

Myths about Pain and Dying

#1—If I take narcotics, I will die as a drug addict.

It is possible to become dependent on narcotics. As I discussed in chapter 4, addiction is different, however. That's the condition where a patient is taking drugs for the euphoric effects, and not for pain relief. There's nothing wrong with being dependent on a narcotic under a doctor's supervision, particularly if you have a terminal illness. The pain patient isn't getting high. No one is breaking the law. If you take narcotics, you won't die as a drug addict. If you don't take narcotics, you may well die in great pain.

Narcotics provide complete pain relief for many terminal illnesses, and they are most effective when doses are slowly increased before the pain gets worse. It is easier to reduce pain before it arrives, as with preemptive analgesia, than to play catch-up and reduce pain after it has settled in. A terminal patient with cancer or HIV or diabetes endures so much pain that there is simply no medication left over to give her a "high."

#2—If I take narcotics, I don't need to take any other medications for pain relief.

Narcotics don't work on all types of pain. Other medications actually have specific effects that you still might need. I once had a patient with prostate cancer that had metastasized throughout his body. We prescribed oral narcotics for pain relief, and increased his dose over time, with great effect. One night, he was stricken by a horrible new pain around his rib cage. We knew that the cancer had already attached to his ribs, but this sharp nerve pain came out of nowhere. The patient mentioned that he had stopped taking Motrin a few days earlier. He had decided that Motrin must be redundant, since he was now taking narcotics. But the nerve pain in his ribs was not affected by the narcotics. After two days of resuming the Motrin, in addition to his narcotics maintenance, the rib pain was gone.

Another cancer patient, Susan D., broke her arm in a car accident. We gave her a cast and a temporary painkiller for the acute pain of her broken bone. Susan decided, on her own, that since she was already taking a long-acting narcotic, she didn't need the new short-acting narcotic painkiller. But each drug was intended to affect a different kind of pain. She endured the pain of a broken arm as if she had taken no pain relief medication at all. This suffering made her despair about the terminal illness, and we had to play catch-up with Susan's cancer pain until it was under control.

#3—I should deal with the pain myself, somehow. It's too embarrassing to complain to my doctor.

This is not a fight with the school yard bully to see if he can make you cry while everyone is watching. Dying is not a test to see how much pain you can endure. There is no reason to be stoic about pain, or to ignore it as if it will go away. It will not go away. Sometimes, patients believe that their doctors know they are in pain, and that the pain is already being treated. These patients believe that they, themselves, are simply not responding correctly to treatment. Describing your pain is not considered complaining, rather it is encouraged. A terminal patient can accomplish many things and enjoy his remaining time with full capacity, if he is not sitting at home in pain.

#4—*The doctor says that pain is simply part of this disease, and there is nothing that can be done about it.*

Some physicians might believe this, because pain is not their specialty. Some doctors downplay this condition in terminal patients. Similarly, a brain surgeon might not care to treat his patient's hypertension—if it's not a surgical problem, then it's not his area of responsibility. Because pain management is still a relatively new field, some physicians are not accustomed to having this specialist involved in a patient's care, or they simply find it easier not to consult yet another specialist. While pain is still a part of many terminal illnesses, there are now many safe options that can eliminate it.

#5—*It's better to stay in bed, because it doesn't hurt as much and then I don't have to take any pain medication.*

I work very hard to overcome this mistaken philosophy in patients. They sometimes undermedicate themselves to the point where they cannot get out of bed because it hurts too much. I sometimes refer to such patients as being in "chalk-line" status—if they lie in a particular position in bed and don't move, then they have no pain. So they keep their body rigid within this imaginary chalk line to prevent pain. I do not think chalk-line pain-free status is a good enough goal for any patient.

By definition, a terminal patient has limited time left. During that time she should be able to do as much as she can to enjoy her life. If this means taking medication to do it, there is no reason not to. Lying around in bed is not the best thing for anyone to do in their last weeks or months. The idea that refusing pain medication is preferable or nobler than taking some will inexplicably confine a patient to her bed, for all her remaining days.

Ninety percent of the pain of any terminal illness can be completely controlled with medications. Although I seem to focus all my attention here on narcotics, they are not the only medications that relieve the pain of terminal patients. Any of the techniques described in this book can be used to make a terminal patient more comfortable. Even aspirin is helpful, and so are nonsteroidal anti-inflammatory drugs. As with any chronic pain, in fact, sometimes those work even better than narcotics. For Nancy D., a seventy-year-old cancer patient, we found that Advil was not effective on her tumor pain, but that Aleve worked very well. After four months, the Aleve was no longer effective, so we moved Nancy on to long-acting OxyContin. This worked well, but I was concerned about the side effects in her particular condition. The OxyContin was sedating, and although Nancy had no pain, she also had very little energy. Within three months, we agreed to implant an intrathecal infusion pump, which enabled us to lower the morphine dose considerably. This did the trick—Nancy even resumed her weekly tennis game. She felt better than she had in a long time, even though her terminal cancer was getting worse. This might seem like a small thing, but to Nancy it made a world of difference.

Palliative Care

Palliative care is the active total care of a patient whose disease is not responsive to curative treatment. Control of pain, of other symptoms, and of psychological, social, and spiritual problems is paramount. The goal of palliative care is achievement of the best possible quality of life for patients and their families. Many aspects of palliative care are also applicable earlier in the course of the illness, in conjunction with anticancer treatment. As defined by the World Health Organization, palliative care:

- affirms life and regards dying as a normal process;
- neither hastens nor postpones death;
- provides relief from pain and other distressing symptoms;
- integrates the psychological and spiritual aspects of patient care;
- offers a support system to help patients live as actively as possible until death;
- offers a support system to help the family cope during the patient's illness and in their own bereavement.

Radiotherapy, chemotherapy, and surgery have a place in palliative care, provided that the symptomatic benefits of treatment clearly outweigh the disadvantages. Investigative procedures are kept to a minimum.

My Definition of Palliative Care

To palliate means to relieve, without curing. Palliative care is not synonymous with pain management—it is its own specialty, encompassing all of a patient's needs on a highly individual basis. Palliative care includes the treatment of terminal disease and also the care of patients with chronic, debilitating diseases that are not necessarily terminal, such as a child with severe birth defects. Many specialists are consulted for someone's palliative care, forming a team under the leadership of the patient's primary-care provider. This team might include specialists from the fields of pain management, oncology, psychiatry, nursing, social services, gerontology, physical therapy, and internal medicine, as well as involving religious support. The team for each patient might be composed differently, but its goal is the same: to provide for every aspect of that patient's ongoing care.

Fred G., a fifty-five-year-old attorney, had lung cancer that had spread to his spinal cord. His oncologist estimated that he had three months to live. When a patient and his family hear news like this, there are many issues that need to be confronted, and no time to lose. Pain management is only one of them. Other issues to be determined might include the extent of treatment, eventual plans for resuscitative efforts, and whether to stay in a hospital or a hospice. Emotional issues about death and dying must be confronted, through either an emotional or spiritual support system. Each specialist in the palliative team contributes when his expertise is required, and then that team member steps aside until his knowledge is needed for another decision down the line. I was called in twice to adjust Fred's pain management, to make sure he was comfortable as well as mentally alert. During this maintenance period, the team might be pared down to the nurse and the primary-care doctor. The goal of palliative care includes not just care of the patient, but the support of the entire family.

It is possible you are reading this and thinking, well, all hospitals provide palliative care. While it is indeed becoming more common, it is not typical to find this sort of team management at any health facility. Most institutions have the array of specialists, but most do not have a system that teams them up to help patients cope with the variety of issues. If you or a loved one have a terminal illness, I encourage you to pursue the palliative care options through your local HMO or hospital.

In his book *How We Die*, Dr. Sherwin Nuland wrote that the greatest dignity to be found in death is the dignity of the life that preceded it. Hope resides in the meaning of what our lives have been. There is no meaning in pain, and patients would no doubt prefer to end their days with dignity rather than battling pain. The entire goal of my practice is to maintain quality of life, or to revive one that was lost, for the living as well as for the dying. Any person with any disease may live life to its fullest, without pain.

CHAPTER 10

Professional Resources and Directories for Finding a Pain-Management Specialist

You cannot resolve chronic pain on your own, not even after reading this book. I wrote *Painbuster* with the intention that you seek professional help to guide you through the Painbuster program. Now, perhaps, your challenge is to find the appropriate specialist near you who will help you implement this program.

There are now almost two thousand pain centers in the United States, and at least three thousand doctors who call themselves specialists in chronic pain. Any physician can call herself a pain-management specialist; there are no restrictions on using that title as a description of one's practice. As I mentioned back in chapter 1, you traditionally had to be a specially trained anesthesiologist in order to achieve board-certification as a pain-management specialist. Since 2000, any physician may now train for, and receive, board-certification in pain management. These might be specialists from psychology, internal medicine, physical medicine, or neurology.

As an anesthesiologist, I naturally tend to consider

that anesthesiologists are the most qualified of pain-management specialists. We can do almost every procedure you might need, plus we have the advantage of being the most experienced at using needles for intricate procedures. However, there is a wide array of other specialists who can help you implement the Painbuster program, including a neurologist, orthopedist, or rheumatologist. You might find a psychologist who is a pain-management specialist, and that doctor might be most helpful. But if you need any special procedures, you might be more comfortable using a doctor who is an anesthesiologist or neurologist.

It would be impossible to list the thousands of resources across the country, but there are a number of organizations that provide names and phone numbers of pain-management specialists in your area. Here is a list of directories for you to consult to locate a good doctor near you.

Where to Find
Pain-Management Specialists

American Academy of Pain Management
13947 Mono Way A
Sonora, CA 95370
Phone: (209) 533-9744
Fax: (209) 533-9750
Web: www.aapainmanage.org

The AAPM Web site lists the names and phone numbers for thousands of pain-management specialists across the country. It is one of the most complete directories available.

The American Chronic Pain Association
P.O. Box 850
Rocklin, CA 95677
Phone: (916) 632-0922
Fax: (916) 632-3208
Web: www.theacpa.org

The American Pain Society
4700 W. Lake Avenue
Glenview, IL 60025
Phone: (847) 375-4715
Fax: (847) 375-6315
Web: www.ampainsoc.org

International Association for the Study of Pain
(IASP)
909 NE 43rd Street, Suite 306
Seattle, WA 98105-6020
Phone: (206) 547-6409
Fax: (206) 547-1703
Web: www.halcyon.com/iasp

The American Pain Foundation
111 S. Calvert Street, Suite 2700
Baltimore, MD 21202
Web: www.painfoundation.org

The National Foundation for the Treatment of Pain
1330 Skyline Drive #21
Monterey, CA 93940
Phone: (831) 655-8812
Fax: (831) 655-2823
Web: www.paincare.org

National Chronic Pain Outreach Association (NCPOA)
7979 Old Georgetown Road, Suite 100
Bethesda, MD 20814-2429
Phone: (301) 652-4948
Fax: (301) 907-0745
Web: www.neurosurgery.mgh.harvard.edu/
NCPAINOA.HTM

American Cancer Society
Offices and resources nationwide
Phone: (800) ACS-2345
Web: www.cancer.org

Cancer Care, Inc.
National Office
275 Seventh Avenue
New York, NY 10001
Phone: (212) 302-2400 or
(800) 813-HOPE (4673)
Web: www.cancercareinc.org

The Arthritis Foundation
National Office
1330 W. Peachtree Street
Atlanta, GA 30309
Phone: (404) 872-7100
Arthritis Answers: (800) 283-7800
Web: www.arthritis.org

The Dannemiller Memorial Educational Foundation
"Triumph Over Pain"
12500 Network Boulevard, Suite 101
San Antonio, TX 78249-3302
Phone: (800) 328-2308
Fax: (210) 641-8329
Web: www.pain.com

The American Society of Regional Anesthesia
and Pain Medicine
1910 Byrd Avenue, Suite 100
P.O. Box 11086
Richmond, VA 23230-1086
Phone: (804) 282-0010
Fax: (804) 282-0090
Web: www.asra.com

Acknowledgments

I am indebted to Dr. John J. Bonica for the inspiration to become a pain-management specialist. I must also acknowledge the long-term support of my colleagues throughout my career, as well as their ideas and the continuous reinforcement of their motivation. I am thankful to the nurses who were an integral part of developing a caring approach to patients, especially Kathleen McMann, R.N., at Walter Reed Army Medical Center, Josephine Musto, R.N., at Saint Vincent's Hospital, Mary Carter, A.N.P., and Elaine Herzog, A.N.P., at North Shore University Hospital.

This book could not have been completed without the superb medical talents of Jeffrey W. Buncher, M.D., and Artur Pacult, M.D., of Charleston, South Carolina. I am also grateful to John Sterling and Deb Brody at Henry Holt and Company, and to Jane O'Boyle, for all the evenings she spent on a cell phone with a tape recorder, interpreting illegible hospital jargon and poor spelling into something that everyone could understand. Janis

Donnaud is the best literary agent there is, and she is also my most persistent patient. If she hadn't had chronic back trouble, this book might never have been written. Some things are a blessing in disguise, Janis. Your pain has helped a lot of other people feel better, too. Thanks, also, to my parents, Milton and Poppy, and to my extended family, for their constant encouragement.

My greatest joys in life are the love and support of my wife, Christine, our daughter, Maria, and our son, Nicholas. Along with them, the greatest lessons in my life have come from my remarkable patients. Their extraordinary determination, patience, and insight continue to teach me new things every day, and to fill me with the satisfaction that hope is not only eternal, but effective. Thank you for letting me come into your lives and for teaching me the value of trust.

Glossary

Definitions of specific ailments can be found in chapter 7: "The A to Z of Chronic Pain Syndromes," on page 149.

ABLATION—the removal of a nerve by one of a variety of surgical methods.

ACETAMINOPHEN—an over-the-counter pain reliever and fever reducer; the generic name for Tylenol.

ACUPUNCTURE—the Chinese medical practice that treats pain by inserting needles into specific sites on the body.

ACUTE PAIN—a sharp or severe "normal" pain, such as from a trauma or injury, that recedes over time.

ANESTHETIC—a substance, such as novocaine or lidocaine, that produces local or general insensibility to pain.

ANTICONVULSANT—a medication that prevents or relieves seizures and muscle contractions.

BENZODIAZEPINE—a pharmaceutical muscle relaxant.

BIOFEEDBACK—a method of electronically monitoring muscle response in physical therapy.

BRETYLIUM BIER BLOCKADE—a local infusion of antiarrhythmic medication to relieve pain.

BUPIVACAINE—a type of local anesthetic.

CAT (COMPUTERIZED AXIAL TOMOGRAPHY) SCAN—a specialized X-ray instrument that displays computerized cross sections of the body, providing visualization of soft tissues such as the brain, lungs, liver, and spleen.

DOUBLE EFFECT—when the side effects of a pain medication, such as slower breathing, make a sick patient more vulnerable than usual.

ENDORPHIN—a group of amino acids in the body that act as natural opiates and raise one's pain threshold.

ENKEPHALIN—one of the amino acids in the body that bind to morphine receptors and temporarily relieve pain through the central nervous system.

EPIDURAL—referring to the lumbar area of the spine, in the space between the spinal cord and the dura.

EPINEPHRINE—a stress-response hormone that increases heart rate and blood pressure, also known as "fight or flight" response.

IBUPROFEN—the generic name for Motrin and Advil, among others, the chemical name of the anti-inflammatory substance most often used to control the pain of arthritis.

INTRATHECAL INFUSION—the surgically implanted pump that delivers pain medication directly to the local area.

ISCHEMIA—local deficiency of blood flow.

LIDOCAINE—a synthetic compound used as a local anesthetic.

LUMBAR—of or pertaining to the area on either side of the spinal column, between the lower ribs and the hipbones, including the lower vertebrae.

MORPHINE—the most important narcotic and principal element of opium, used as a pain reliever.

MRI (MAGNETIC RESONANCE IMAGING)—a noninvasive test using magnetic and radio waves to display computer-generated sectional images of the body and its internal structure.

MULTIDISCIPLINARY—combining several separate branches of learning or expertise.

MYOFASCIAL PAIN—muscle and soft tissue pain.

NARCOTIC—a class of substances that blunts the senses and relieves pain, such as opium, morphine, and alcohol. In large doses, a narcotic might produce euphoria and, when used constantly, can cause addiction.

NEURALGIA—sharp pain along the course of a nerve.

NEURITIS—inflammation, or swelling, of a nerve.

NEUROTRANSMITTER—any of several chemical substances, such as epinephrine, that transmit nerve impulses.

NONSTEROIDAL ANTI-INFLAMMATORY DRUG (NSAID)—a pharmaceutical substance, such as ibuprofen, that acts like a steroid to reduce inflammation.

NOREPINEPHRINE—a neurotransmitter that constricts blood vessels and raises blood pressure.

OPIATE—a narcotic drug containing opium or its derivatives.

OPIOID—any opium-like substance, whether natural (such as endorphins) or synthetic (such as methadone).

PCA (PATIENT-CONTROLLED ANALGESIA)—an intravenous device that allows the patient to deliver her own pain medication when she needs it, within limits.

PERIPHERAL NERVES—the sensory nerves throughout the body, excluding the ones in the spinal cord and brain.

PLACEBO—a substance having no pharmacological effect but given to satisfy a patient who supposes it to be a medication, sometimes used as a control device in drug experiments. Also known as a "sugar pill."

RADICULOPATHY—pain in the roots of a nerve.

STEROID—any of a large group of fat-soluble organic compounds that affect the body, such as bile acids and sex hormones.

SYMPATHETIC NERVOUS SYSTEM—nerves that arise from the lumbar and thoracic regions of the spinal cord and that encompass the "involuntary" nerves such as heartbeat, pupil dilation, etc.

TENS (TRANSCUTANEOUS ELECTRICAL NERVE STIMULATION)—a self-operated portable device that sends electrical impulses to areas of chronic pain, through electrodes placed on the skin.

TRIGGER POINT—the local injured area of the body where a slight stimulus causes severe pain.

VASCULAR—pertaining to ducts that convey fluids, such as blood vessels.

VISCERAL—pertaining to the organs in the cavities of the body, especially in the abdominal cavity, such as the intestines and the bowel.

Index

About the Authors

JOHN M. STAMATOS, M.D., is the medical director of North Shore Pain Services in Long Island, New York, and codirector of the Cohn Pain Management Center of the North Shore University/Long Island Jewish Health Care System. A graduate of Walter Reed Army Medical Center in Washington, D.C., he spent several years as a pain-management specialist at Saint Vincent's Hospital in New York City.

JANE O'BOYLE is a writer who lives in Charleston, South Carolina.